LOOK TO YOUR HEALTH

LOOK TO YOUR HEALTH

What You Should Know About
the Body,
Common Diseases,
and
Healthful Living

Herbert M. Dean, M.D.
John J. Massarelli, M.D.

VNR VAN NOSTRAND REINHOLD COMPANY
New York   Cincinnati   Toronto   London   Melbourne

Art, excluding pages 35, 36, and 178, by Radu Vero.

Published by Van Nostrand Reinhold Company
A division of Litton Educational Publishing, Inc.
135 West 50th Street, New York, NY 10020, U.S.A.

Van Nostrand Reinhold Limited
1410 Birchmount Road
Scarborough, Ontario M1P 2E7, Canada

Van Nostrand Reinhold Australia Pty. Ltd.
17 Queen Street
Mitcham, Victoria 3132, Australia

Van Nostrand Reinhold Company Limited
Molly Millars Lane
Wokingham, Berkshire, England

16 15 14 13 12 11 10 9 8 7 6 5 4 3 2 1

Library of Congress Cataloging in Publication Data

Dean, Herbert M.
  Look to your health.

  Includes index.
    1. Medicine, Popular. 2. Health. I. Massarelli,
John, joint author. II. Title. [DNLM: 1. Medicine—
Popular works. 2. Patients—Education. WB120.3 D281L]
RC81.D285   616   79-22833
ISBN 0-442-24742-7

We dedicate this book to our wives, Vera and Joan, to our good friend, Neil Heffernan, Jr., and to our colleagues and patients at the Fallon Clinic.

CONTENTS

Foreword

We wrote this book because there are a lot of people who need the information it contains about health and disease.

In our practice we often see people who could have avoided unnecessary suffering, disability, and expense if they had gone to the doctor sooner. Literally daily, we see people who don't need a doctor at all, but who think they do because of a trivial symptom or condition which will disappear without treatment, or because of something that is not disease at all. Many of our patients worry unnecessarily over illnesses that need not be a major concern if only they knew more about them. Most importantly, there are many chronic diseases that the patient must know about so that he can participate effectively in his own treatment. Too often, patients with diabetes or arthritis or hypertension fail to do as well as they should because they do not understand enough about their own disease to take care of themselves properly.

Sometimes their condition is not cured or patients do not do as well as they should because they fail to follow the prescribed treatment. There are several reasons for this behavior. It is only natural to stop taking a drug when you feel better and the reason for taking it has seemingly disappeared. There are many circumstances, however, when such action is unwise. Persons with a sore throat caused by the streptococcus germ, a bacterial pneumonia, or similar acute infections may begin to feel better long before the germ that causes their sickness is completely eradicated. Premature discontinuance of an antibiotic may only result in a flare-up of their disease later. The full amount of medicine prescribed is necessary for complete cure. A similar situation exists in some chronic diseases such as high blood pressure and diabetes, where symptoms occur only late, or after complications have developed, but where proper treatment can control the basic condition and often prevent serious problems. Other reasons for non-compliance or failure to follow the prescribed treatment are more difficult for most of us to understand. These include going on a vacation (sickness never takes a day off!), running out of a prescription that should be refilled, moving away from the doctor's or pharmacist's neighborhood, and even getting mad at the doctor!

We think doctors have a major responsibility in many cases

where non-compliance has been a factor in treatment failure. The patient must be informed as to why he's taking the medicine, or is on the diet, or doing the exercises, so that he or she knows exactly what is being prescribed, why, and for how long. In addition to imparting information, this educational process also helps motivate people to cooperate in their own medical care. In persons with chronic diseases, education must be repeated periodically to reinforce their desire to do what is proper for their health. Patient education is important for patient compliance.

*   *   *

Doctors recognize that teaching patients about their condition is part of therapy. Unfortunately, they simply cannot educate every patient to the extent they would like.

Consider the circumstances in which physician-patient education is carried out. First of all, the physical setting—usually a small, functionally furnished examining room—is strange and intimidating. Secondly, the doctor is pressed for time, and both he and the patient are aware of the full waiting room or the late hour.

There is a language barrier, for the technical terms which flow so easily from the doctor's tongue are incomprehensible to most people, and in fact their very sound sometimes seems calculated to instill fear. For example, "osteoarthritis of the cervical spine" can augur a long-term, painful, crippling, hopeless disease to the patient, when it may mean nothing more to the doctor than a little bone spur in the neck. Many of those glib phrases which satisfy some persons ("upside-down stomach" for diaphragmatic hiatus hernia, or "white cells eating up the red cells" for leukemia, or "gland trouble" for we don't know what) do not adequately explain what is wrong.

Finally, there probably is no worse time for a person to learn anything than when he has just been told his own diagnosis. His emotional state is a cacophony: *anxiety* that he has the disease, *fear* of pain or not being able to live normally, *relief* that he does not have the quickly fatal cancer or heart disease he thought he'd had, sometimes *anger* that he is not perfectly well while his overweight, cigarette-puffing brother-in-law is, and so forth.

Attempts at education under all these handicaps usually do not succeed, and the patient is going to have to settle for answers to specific questions he asks on subsequent visits.

*   *   *

Of course, the average person cannot be expected to know as much about his body and the things that can go wrong with it as a trained physician. But there is no excuse for anyone not knowing some basic facts about the symptoms of common diseases that require medical attention, about the course of common diseases, and about healthful ways of living. We hope our book will prove to be a source of this information.

H.M.D. and J.J.M.

About the Authors

Doctors Herbert M. Dean and John J. Massarelli are in the full-time private practice of internal medicine at the Fallon Clinic, a multi-specialty group practice in Worcester, Massachusetts. Together they have spent over 30 years in caring for patients, and have written this health book for the concerned person based on their practice experience.

Dr. Massarelli is certified as a specialist by the American Board of Internal Medicine. His training included a fellowship at the Mayo Clinic, where he earned a Master of Science degree in Internal Medicine. He is a past president of the Massachusetts Society of Internal Medicine, and a former editor of the *Worcester District Medical News*. Many physicians and their families are among his patients, and he is often consulted by other doctors in difficult medical cases.

Dr. Dean is one of a very small group of doctors who are certified in three different specialties: Internal Medicine, Hematology (blood diseases), and Medical Oncology (cancer treatment). Dr. Dean's depth of experience in caring for terminally ill patients has endowed him with a compassion for which he is known by many referring doctors. He is a student of medical history, and a collector of old medical books.

Both authors are on the faculty of The University of Massachusetts Medical School and are active in teaching medical students and physicians in training. They are Fellows of the American College of Physicians and belong to many medical and professional organizations. They have written articles in leading medical journals.

LOOK TO YOUR HEALTH

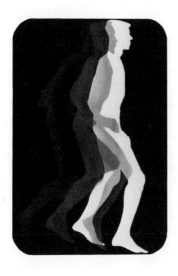

An Ounce of Prevention

A search for ways to remain youthful despite advancing years has concerned people in every generation. Ponce de Leon trudged through Florida searching for the waters of the "Fountain of Youth." Nowadays people consume large quantities of vitamins, hormones, and "health foods," partly in the hope of preventing degenerative processes and of growing older without showing the signs of age.

From time to time, someone discovers groups of people residing in an isolated part of the world where many of their numbers live well past a hundred years. Efforts to find *the* factor responsible for their longevity always meet with failure. One such group, reported recently as "Shangri-La in Ecuador," had a score of persons older than 100 years, who appeared younger than their chronological age, were quite active, and had remained mentally alert. These people seldom develop malignant tumors or arteriosclerosis. Although their diet is largely a vegetarian one of about 1,700 calories a day, they may smoke 40 or more cigarettes a day and drink two to four cups of rum. Other similar long-lived groups reside in Kashmair, and in Abkhalia in the Soviet Union.

No uniform diet pattern, ancestry, or climate can be found

to explain these remarkable clusters of individuals. Commonly, most of these centenarians who have been studied have parents who lived to ripe old ages. Perhaps the secret of their youthfulness includes the combination of good genes, the physical activity inherent in a rural setting, the tranquility provided by isolation from the pressures of contemporary life, and freedom from environmental pollution.

Now consider these simple, commonsense rules of good health: (a) three meals daily, with special emphasis on breakfast, (b) moderate body weight, (c) seven or eight hours of sleep per night, (d) moderate exercise, (e) moderate use of alcohol, and (f) no smoking. A recent study of 7,000 persons demonstrated an amazing conclusion about these health habits: a 45-year-old man who lives by three or fewer of these rules can expect to live to be 67, but one who observes all of them has a life expectancy of 78, an eleven-year advantage!

Imagine what price you could command for an elixir that would enable a middle-aged person to add eleven years to his life. Yet here is a free regimen of easily followed guidelines which would be just that, and which are so often ignored.

That wise old fisherman of the seventeenth century, Isaak Walton, said, "Look to your health; if you have it, praise God and value it next to a good conscience; for health is the second blessing that we mortals are capable of—a blessing that money cannot buy; therefore, value it and be thankful for it."

Most of this book deals with disease, the opposite of health. In reading it you will learn about most of the things that can go wrong with your health, and what you can do to correct these things. This chapter will try to tell you how to "look to your health." We will consider diet in some detail, then discuss two common health hazards: obesity and cigarette smoking, and then tell you about exercise and health. Finally, periodic health examination will be considered.

The Normal Diet

To define a "normal diet" is really impossible, because of the enormous diversity in tastes and taboos from one culture to another, in the availability of different foods in various places, and in what foods people can afford to buy. The choice of our menu largely reflects personal likes and dislikes, built on national, cultural, and religious factors, and the food actually put on the table in most households is largely determined by monetary considerations.

The diet of an average American is considerably different from that of an Australian Bushman, a Sudanese farmer, a Peruvian goatherd, or a Japanese fisherman. Yet in each of these cases the individual's diet may provide for his nutritional requirements so that he maintains a healthy body. For most Americans, meats such as beef, chicken, lamb or pork, as well as cheeses, eggs, and milk products provide most of the protein we need. In other countries, the sources of protein may be soybeans, fish, snails, snakes, locusts, or meat from dogs and horses.

The energy supplied by any food is measured in units called *calories*, and is equivalent to the amount of heat that food can supply as it is burned up. Three classes of food supply the energy and the building material for our bodies: protein, fats, and carbohydrates. One gram of protein or carbohydrate furnishes four calories; a gram of fat yields nine calories. Pregnant women and growing children require more calories than the average adult, men burn more food energy than women, and big people more than little people. The amount of exercise performed each day is the major determining factor in how many calories of energy are used up, and, therefore, must be made up by food intake. A 45-year-old woman who works as a typist and who weighs 116 pounds may require 1,900 calories daily, while a professional football player in training camp needs over 6,000 calories every day.

Protein, as we have seen above, is generally obtained from animal products. Nutritionists have determined that human beings require at least 0.5 gram, and preferably 1 to 1.5 grams of protein in the daily diet for every kilogram of weight. This means that a 70 kilogram (150 pound) person should eat between 70 grams (2.3 ounces) and 105 grams (3.5 ounces) of protein every day. The carbohydrates in our diet are in the starches, sugar, fruits, and milk we eat. About one-half or a little less than half of our total caloric intake is in the form of carbohydrates. Fats in the average American diet contribute about one-third of the day's calories.

Besides these three classes of foods, we also need small amounts of certain minerals and vitamins, which do not provide fuel for energy, and so have no caloric value. The minerals include iron, calcium, phosphorus, iodine, and magnesium.

The consumer has become health food and vitamin oriented. To meet this new interest there has been a surge in the available number of health products and stores selling various "health and natural foods." There are many combinations and dosages of various vitamins for sale with claims for their effectiveness in preserving good health and in controlling degenerative diseases and the aging process. Those who are pushing special foods or vitamins derived from natural sources as opposed to synthetic sources preach the benefits and superiority of their products and imply potential hazards of many conventional food products that contain various additives and preservatives. These claims and counterclaims only confuse the average person. The role of vitamins in maintaining health and the consequences of vitamin deficiency as well as nutritional sources of vitamins will be highlighted in this chapter.

Vitamins

Casimir Funk coined the term "vitamin" in 1912, believing that various disorders were caused by the lack of certain essential proteins. Even though the chemical identification of the missing vitamins in various diseases took place only during the past 50 years, the diseases caused by vitamin deficiencies have been known for thousands of years. Scurvy, the lack of vitamin C, was described in the Ebers Papyrus from Egypt. Nicholas Tulp, the great Dutch anatomist made famous in a painting by Rembrandt, described beriberi, a disorder due to lack of vitamin B_1. Vitamins are usually divided into the fat-soluble group (A, D, E, and K) and the water-soluble group (B complex, C). The fat-soluble vitamins are less likely to be lost in cooking or processing than the water-soluble group. The fat-soluble vitamins are stored in the body, so that large doses of them may cause toxic symptoms.

 Vitamin A is derived from our foods usually in the form of B-carotene and is stored in our liver. The vitamin is found in milk, butter, egg yolk, and the green leaves of plants including broccoli, spinach, and escarole, as well as carrots and fruits. The activity of the vitamin is not reduced by ordinary cooking or boiling of food but may be destroyed by ultraviolet light. One ounce of butter provides approximately 1,200 IU (International Units), one quart of milk 1,400 IU, carrots 2,200-47,000 IU per 100 grams, and leafy vegetables 6,000 to 12,000 IU per 100 grams.

 Vitamin A deficiency can occur because of dietary lack, improper absorption of vitamin A due to bowel diseases

United States Food and Drug Administration Recommended Daily Needs

	Unit	Infants (0-12 mo.)	Children under 4 years	Adults & Children 4 or more years	Pregnant or Lactating Women
Vitamin A	IU	1500	2500	5000	8000
Vitamin D	IU	400	400	400	400
Vitamin E	IU	5	10	30	30
Vitamin C	Mg	35	40	60	60
Folic Acid	Mg	0.1	0.2	0.4	0.8
Thiamine (B$_1$)	Mg	0.5	0.7	1.5	1.7
Riboflavin (B$_2$)	Mg	0.6	0.8	1.7	2.0
Niacin	Mg	8	9	20	20
Vitamin B$_6$	Mg	0.4	0.7	2	2.5
Vitamin B$_{12}$	Mcg	2	3	6	8
Biotin	Mg	0.05	0.15	0.3	0.3
Pantothenic acid	Mg	3	5	10	10
Calcium	G	0.6	0.8	1	1.3
Phosphorus	G	0.5	0.8	1	1.3
Iodine	Mcg	45	70	150	150
Iron	Mg	15	10	18	18
Magnesium	Mg	70	200	400	450
Copper	Mg	0.6	1	2	2
Zinc	Mg	5	8	15	15

IU = International Units
Mg = Milligram
Mcg = Microgram
G = Gram

(celiac disease, sprue, or inflammatory bowel disease), or thyroid disease (since thyroid hormone is necessary to convert the vitamin precursor, carotene, to Vitamin A in the liver).

In vitamin A deficiency, nerve cells in the retina of the eye, called rods, do not function properly, causing night blindness, which is inability to see in dim light. Other areas of the eye become affected as well, causing drying and wrinkling of the conjunctiva (the membrane that lines the eyelid and covers the front part of the eyeball) with infection or ulceration and softening of the cornea, eventually leading to perforation and blindness.

The skin also may be involved in vitamin A deficiency, with dryness, roughness, and itching.

Excess vitamin A, almost always due to overuse of vitamin

A tablets, causes loss of appetite, irritability, headache, hair loss and dry skin, enlargement of the liver and spleen, increased pressure on the brain, increased levels of blood calcium, and growth retardation in children.

Vitamin D is necessary for the formation and maintenance of normal bone. This vitamin influences the absorption of calcium and phosphorus from the intestine. There are several forms of vitamin D. Ergocalciferol (vitamin D_2) comes from plants and is the active ingredient in most vitamin D preparations. Cholecalciferol (vitamin D_3) is the "natural" human vitamin, since it is made by the skin from 7-dehydrocholesterol in the presence of ultraviolet light (sunlight), and is also available in our diet from animal sources—milk, egg yolk, and fish oils. Within the body, the liver and kidneys convert vitamin D_3 into more active forms.

The vitamin D content of fresh milk is 100 IU per quart and that of butter 10 to 100 IU per ounce. The vitamin D content of food products depends on the season of the year—it is higher in summer than in winter. Vegetable oils and margarines contain little vitamin D. Most commercial homogenized milk has been fortified to provide 400 IU of vitamin D per quart.

Vitamin D deficiency occurs because of inadequate dietary intake or lack of exposure to sunlight. Since vitamin D is fat soluble, any process that interferes with the absorption of fat by the intestine can cause a deficiency.

Rickets, a disease occurring in infancy and early childhood (after six months of age) is caused by vitamin D deficiency. In the absence of vitamin D a calcium deficiency occurs; normal calcification of growing cartilage fails to take place, producing skeletal deformities involving the ribs, the legs, and the skull, causing permanently retarded growth. In adults, a disease called osteomalacia develops with vitamin D deficiency. The blood levels of calcium and phosphorus are reduced and may cause tetany, cramps of various muscle groups. The skeletal bone becomes depleted of calcium, and bone pain and fractures may develop.

Excessive intake of vitamin D for prolonged periods of time causes abnormal amounts of calcium in the blood, leading to lack of appetite, nausea and vomiting, weakness, excessive thirst, constipation, drowsiness, elevated blood pressure, and in time calcium deposits in blood vessels and subcutaneous tissue, kidney stones, kidney failure, and, finally, death.

There is no evidence that healthy, active adults require

supplemental vitamin D unless they are never exposed to sunlight (coal miners working the first shift, for example).

Vitamin E has been hailed as the miracle vitamin, despite our lack of knowledge about the biochemical function of this vitamin in man. A fat-soluble substance called tocopherol, meaning to bring childbirth, was initially identified as necessary for reproduction in rats. Since it can take up oxygen, vitamin E protects other compounds such as unsaturated fatty acids and other oxygen-sensitive substances such as vitamin A and vitamin C from oxidation.

Vegetable oils—corn, sugar, peanut, or coconut, and vegetables, fruits, and grain products contain significant quantities of vitamin E.

Vitamin E deficiency may occur in illnesses associated with faulty absorption of dietary fats or with excessive use of mineral oil. The requirement of vitamin E increases with the dietary intake of unsaturated fatty acids.

In adults, no disorder following vitamin E deficiency has been actually proved, despite a wide variety of disease patterns caused by vitamin E deficiency in animals. The vitamin has no effectiveness in the treatment of sterility, neuromuscular disorders, graying of hair, or cardiovascular diseases. Vitamin E is effective only in preventing vitamin E deficiency.

Recently, a need for vitamin E in premature infants was recognized because it was found that hemolytic anemia was cured by vitamin E. Newborn infants fed a diet high in polyunsaturated fatty acids develop body swelling, irritability, and skin changes, and these are corrected by vitamin E. Large doses of vitamin E, in excess of 800 IU, have caused intestinal symptoms, muscle weakness, and disturbances of reproductive functions.

Vitamin K (from the German word koagulation—clotting vitamin) is important in producing certain normal blood-clotting factors in the liver.

The vitamin is present in leafy vegetables and is also synthesized by many species of bacteria which are normally found in the human intestine.

Vitamin K deficiency can occur after prolonged use of antibiotics which destroy intestinal bacteria or any illness that interferes with the absorption of this fat soluble vitamin—disease of the bile ducts or malabsorption states. The commonest cause of vitamin K deficiency is the use of an anticoagulant drug such as Coumadin, which prevents clotting by acting as a vitamin K antagonist (nullifying the action of vitamin K).

Thiamine, vitamin B_1, is present in fresh green vegetables, whole cereals, yeast, liver, and pork. Poor sources of vitamin B_1 include human milk, nonenriched flour, rice, and processed cereals.

Deficiency of vitamin B_1 causes several disorders, including beriberi, Wernicke's encephalopathy, and Korsakoff's psychosis. An official of the Japanese Navy discovered beriberi could be cured by decreasing the rice diet and adding barley, vegetables, meat, and condensed milk.

Beriberi occurs in two forms—wet and dry. Wet beriberi is characterized by massive edema or swelling accompanied by congestive heart failure; in dry beriberi, peripheral neuropathy—numbness and tingling of the lower extremities—is the chief finding. This condition was common among prisoners of the Japanese during World War II.

Wernicke's encephalopathy and Korsakoff's psychosis occur chiefly in alcoholics, who develop confusion, paralysis of the eye muscles, unsteadiness of gait, and peripheral neuropathy. Characteristic brain lesions develop in these conditions. Often these disorders are accompanied by other vitamin B complex deficiencies besides thiamine. Dramatic improvement of some symptoms can follow replacement of thiamine.

Riboflavin, vitamin B_2, is necessary for many reactions in living cells. The vitamin is present in most foods, and especially in dairy and meat items.

A lack of riboflavin is associated with cracking around the mouth, soreness of the tongue, seborrheic dermatitis especially around the nose, and vascularity of the cornea.

Niacin (nicotinic acid) is essential for several important body enzymes. A deficiency of niacin leads to a disorder called pellagra, which is characterized by the three D's: dermatitis, a skin rash especially on the parts of the skin exposed to sunlight; diarrhea; and a dementia, consisting of hallucinations and irritability.

Pellagra is commonly seen in poverty areas of the world where the diet is poor, consisting chiefly of corn. Corn has a very low content of niacin as well as an essential protein builder, tryptophan. As with thiamine deficiency, other vitamin B group deficiencies may coexist in niacin deficiency. In 1935, 3,500 people died of pellagra in the United States. This disease has now virtually disappeared in this country because of improved dietary standards and enrichment of wheat flour. Large doses of nicotinic acid can reduce the level of cholesterol in the blood, and this vitamin has been used in treating atherosclerosis.

Large doses of niacin can cause jaundice, which disappears when the drug is discontinued.

Pantothenic Acid is found in meat, liver, cereals, milk, and vegetables and is also synthesized by intestinal bacteria. It is necessary for reactions in the body involving coenzyme A.

Pantothenic acid deficiency has been induced in volunteers maintained on a restricted diet. Muscle cramps, numbness of the extremities, and impairment of coordination and movement developed. Even though this vitamin plays an important role in human nutrition, it is most unlikely that deficiency occurs except in the most unusual circumstances.

Pyridoxine, vitamin B_6, is present in a wide range of foods including dairy products, meat, cereals and grains, fruits, and vegetables. The vitamin is necessary for many important body reactions.

Vitamin B_6 deficiency may cause a seborrheic rash over the eyes, nose, and mouth, fissures (cracks) and sores around the angles of the mouth, soreness of the tongue, and a neuritis. An unusual type of anemia may respond to treatment with large doses of pyridoxine. Patients with tuberculosis who receive the drug isoniazid may develop a peripheral neuritis (inflammation of the nerves in the feet), which is reversible or preventable by treatment with pyridoxine.

Folic Acid is widely distributed in most plants, but especially green, leafy vegetables, and in liver. It is an important biological catalyst necessary for the transfer of single carbon units.

A healthy person has 50 to 100 times the daily requirement of the vitamin stored in the body, mainly in the liver. A deficiency occurs in patients who are chronically ill and eating poorly, in alcoholics who eat poorly, or in pregnancy, where the daily need increases and may not be met by adequate nutrition. Uncommon causes include malabsorption disorders of the bowel and hemolytic anemia, which increase the body's requirement. A rare cause of folic acid deficiency occurs in infants fed goat's milk, which has a very low content of folic acid.

Folic acid deficiency causes a striking anemia with production of very abnormal-appearing red blood cells and white blood cells. Fissures occur at the angles of the mouth and soreness of the tongue is commonly present as well. Treatment with folic acid rapidly corrects the disturbance.

Vitamin B_{12}, the anti-pernicious anemia factor, occurs in protein foods of animal origin (liver, meat, milk) and requires the presence of a protein màde in the stomach, called intrinsic factor, to allow Vitamin B_{12} to be absorbed from the intestinal tract.

Pernicious anemia is due to an absence of intrinsic factor thereby preventing the absorption of vitamin B_{12}. Vitamin B_{12} deficiency may also occur in strict vegetarians who eat no animal protein; following complete removal of the stomach, which removes the source of intrinsic factor; and in intestinal malabsorption disorders. Vitamin B_{12} deficiency causes an anemia indistinguishable from folic acid deficiency. In time, spinal cord damage occurs, causing numbness of the toes and fingers and eventually muscle weakness. Elderly patients may develop a psychosis, dullness, and overall apathy.

Monthly injections of Vitamin B_{12} correct the anemia, but if the illness has been present long enough to produce overt neurological disease, permanent spinal cord damage may occur.

Ascorbic acid or *vitamin C* is found in most fresh fruits and vegetables, especially citrus fruits and tomatoes. Meats, cereals, and dairy products contain small amounts. The vitamin C content is reduced by approximately 50 percent by boiling, steaming, or microwave cooking. Steam tables used in restaurants destroy much of the vitamin.

Vitamin C deficiency, or scurvy, causes defects in body tissues and in the orderly cónversion of cartilage into bone. Disease occurs in growing bone, teeth, blood vessels, and fibrous tissue. Wounds heal poorly. Early symptoms of vitamin C deficiency include weakness, easy fatigue, and aching of bones, joints, and muscles. The skin becomes dry, rough, and brown. The hairs of the legs and buttock areas become fragmented and coiled, with thickening of the hair follicle. Hemorrhages develop around the hair follicle. Easy bruisability develops, followed by spontaneous hemorrhages into the skin, muscles, and joints. The gums become swollen, boggy, inflamed, and friable. The teeth become loose and fall out.

Treatment of scurvy involves giving ascorbic acid. Lind in England prevented scurvy in British sailors by giving them limes to suck—hence the nickname "Limeys" for British sailors. Scurvy in adults is seldom seen except in food faddists who do not eat fresh fruits and vegetables or who prepare them so as to reduce their vitamin C content.

More recently, large doses of ascorbic acid have been touted as preventing colds. Although a certain degree of skepticism remains regarding their effectiveness, a recent study indicates that vitamin C does not reduce the number of colds but decreases the morbidity of the illness (the length of illness and recovery time from the cold). However, toxic effects are possible with very large doses, so a physician's advice should be sought before taking them.

Biotin is a vitamin B complex present in nearly all foods and bacteria. The vitamin can be inactivated by a diet high in eggwhite. Volunteers made deficient in biotin, after several weeks, developed depression, lassitude, sleepiness, muscle aches, dermatitis, and an anemia which was reversed after treatment with biotin.

The average healthy American adult consuming a typical balanced and varied diet requires no vitamin supplements. Vitamins are useful in growing children, whose requirements may not be met by marginal diets, and during pregnancy, when vitamin needs are increased. Persons with chronic illnesses often have an inadequate dietary intake and benefit from vitamin supplements. A multivitamin containing the recommended doses of the various vitamins is adequate. Excess vitamin consumption serves no purpose except to risk serious side effects.

Minerals

Calcium and Phosphorus.   The bones of our body contain 99 percent of all the body calcium and approximately 75 percent of the body phosphorus.

The need for calcium in the diet is increased during growth spurts in children, especially during infancy and at puberty. Calcium need is increased during pregnancy and breast feeding.

In the section above, the role of vitamin D in calcium absorption as well as disturbances in health caused by excess or deficiency of body calcium levels was described. Although one can get the necessary daily calcium requirement by drinking two cups (one pint) of milk a day, it is one of the nutrients most likely to be at inadequate levels in the average diet.

Phosphorus is present in adequate amounts in most human diets, so that a deficiency state seldom occurs. The mineral plays a major role in many important metabolic processes. Combined with nucleoproteins, phosphorus serves as a constituent of substances important in cell division and transmission of genetic material. The energy for internal cell reactions is provided by high energy phosphorus-containing compounds. Phosphorus is linked to fat substances, producing another class of important compounds called phospholipids.

In the section on anemia the importance of iron, its source, and daily requirement are discussed. The role of iodine is detailed in the section on thyroid diseases.

The trace metals, which include zinc, copper, manganese, chromium, and other minerals, play significant roles in many body enzyme reactions, but are required in very small concentrations and seldom produce medical problems in man.

Vegetarian Diet

Various types of vegetarian diets are popular today. True vegetarians eat food exclusively derived from plants. Lactovegetarians add dairy products to their diet, and lactoovovegetarians eat eggs as well. The less restrictive a vegetarian-type diet, the more likely it is that an individual's dietary requirements will be satisfied.

Protein derived from plant sources tends to be of lower quality than animal-derived protein. Protein supplied by legumes (peas, dried beans) is low in one of the amino acids, methionine, an essential component of human protein, and cereal grains are low in another amino acid, lysine. Animal protein contains the eight essential amino acids—essential in this sense means it must be taken in as food because the human body cannot manufacture it—in available forms and optimal amounts. Mixing legumes with cereal grains provides a better quality protein source than that derived from either alone. By combining foods of plant origin, the needed nutritional protein values supplied by animal sources can be met.

Vitamin B_{12} is lacking in plant-derived foods but is present in eggs and milk. A total vegetarian must add a B_{12}-containing vitamin to his diet or drink fortified soybean milk. Soybeans are used to prepare dishes which taste like animal protein foods and are rich in the B vitamins and iron. Nuts and peanut butter also supply protein. Grains furnish carbohydrates, protein, iron, thiamine, and trace metals. Green leafy vegetables provide riboflavin, calcium, and vitamin A precursors.

All of our nutritional requirements except vitamin B_{12} can be satisfied by a vegetarian-type diet. When food products of animal origin are excluded, greater attention to dietary planning is necessary in order to provide proper nutrition.

Food Additives

Most of us depend on food purchased at supermarkets, where over 30,000 food products are available. More and more of our dietary intake consists of processed, packaged foodstuffs and convenience-type foods (TV dinners, frozen foods, etc.) rather than fresh produce. At different stages of production, pesticides, fertilizers, and food additives are used by the various parts of the food industry.

Approximately a billion pounds of chemicals are used by the food industry to process various food items—five pounds per person per year. A food additive is defined by the Food Production Committee of the National Research Council as a "substance or mixture of substances other than a basic foodstuff which is present in food as a result of any aspect of production, processing, storage or packaging." Food additives serve various functions, including sweetening, acidifying, coloring, flavoring, preserving, thickening, and emulsifying.

As consumers, we rely on the purity and wholesomeness of our food through regulations and enforcement by various local, state, and federal agencies, including the Food and Drug Administration and the Department of Agriculture. Much of the improvement in public health in this country during the last fifty years is a result of the food fortification program with minerals and vitamins. Substantial health benefits have occurred because of enrichment of flour and bread products.

Despite these benefits, genuine concern exists regarding the safety of food prepared with numerous food additives. One has only to check labels to discover the many and various chemical additives. The chief possible adverse effects include inducing cancer (carcinogenic) or causing mutations (genetic changes) in future generations of people.

Although they pose real ecological problems, the use of various chemicals and pesticides is necessary in modern agriculture for control of insects and rodents and to allow for maximal yields in food production. Several years ago, a public fear of consuming cranberries caused widescale abandonment of this fruit from its place at the traditional Thanksgiving feast. A pesticide, aminotriasole, with potential cancer-inducing effects, contaminated part of the cranberry crop because growers did not follow the manufacturers' directions and applied the chemical for weed control before the harvest and not afterward.

Chemicals including hormones and antibiotics have been used in the meat and poultry industry to promote rapid growth and meat content of animals. The safety of the estrogen-containing hormones has been questioned in cattle growing and their use suspended. In general, chemicals may be used in livestock and poultry provided there is no accumulation in milk or significant quantities in the tissues of the animal or its products (eggs).

Similar concerns exist about the dangers of radioactive fallout and the impact on our water supply, agricultural products, and livestock. Contamination of our food supply by radioactive substances such as strontium 90 and cesium 137 has led to monitoring of their levels in various foodstuffs.

Federal laws are supposed to control the safety of various additives before they can be used in food shipped across the country. In general, tests are done that establish the safety of the chemicals when consumed by laboratory animals in doses one hundred times the usual human level.

The original list of substances that could be used in food production or packaging consisted largely of nutrients—vitamins and minerals; subsequent additions have included anticaking agents, stabilizers, spices, natural seasonings, and flavorings, preservatives, and emulsifying agents. Currently more than 500 food additives are generally recognized as safe and allowable for use by the Federal Drug Administration (FDA). Critics of the FDA list for additives point to the large number of approved substances which achieved their status under a "grandfather" clause at the initial formulation of the list—they had been used for many years and were generally considered to be safe. In addition, certain dyes, preservatives, and coloring agents called permissible for use are now felt to be potentially dangerous and their safety not firmly established. Cyclamates, which are no longer permitted as a substitute for sugar because they are a suspected carcinogen, were permitted on the 1969 FDA list. Recent studies have raised the possibility that using saccharine may also cause cancer of the bladder under experimental conditions.

Food Colorings. Most food colorings are derived from coal

tar dyes—one of the earliest known cancer-inducing substances. Many dyes have been banned since 1919, and the list grows larger. In 1960, FDC orange Number 2, and red Number 1 were no longer permitted for use because of deleterious effects, including cancer induction in animals. FDC red Number 4 was restricted to coloring of maraschino cherries and pill coatings because of injury to the adrenal glands of experimental animals. Citrus red Number 2 is now restricted to dye oranges, and yellow Numbers 1, 2, 3, and 4 are no longer allowed because of harmful effects on animals.

The most widely used coal tar dye is red Number 2, which gives a cherry color to products including beverages, ice cream, candies, baked goods, and sausage meat. This coloring has been banned in Russia because of reports of birth defects and cancer in rats, but the results appear unreliable and have not been confirmed in studies done in this country.

Food colorings are not always identified on labels and may appear as "artificial coloring" or "certified color added." The use of certain food additives can be criticized when their purpose is examined. Is it really necessary to color certain food items to make them more appealing to the consumer?

Monosodium Glutamate (MSG). Monosodium glutamate originated in Japan and is a common additive in many food products because of its ability to enhance the taste of foods. The seasoning *Accent* contains MSG.

Many persons are aware of a group of symptoms especially during meals in Chinese restaurants, where MSG is greatly used. The symptoms include chest tightness, headaches, and a burning sensation in the neck and arms. These symptoms are caused by MSG, and this condition is nicknamed the Chinese restaurant syndrome.

Some investigators have reported brain damage in infant mice, rats, and monkeys given MSG, and baby food manufacturers have removed this additive from baby food.

Nitrites. Nitrites are used as preservatives, colorings, and flavorings. The bright pink color of ham, bacon, hot dogs, and cold cuts is derived from them. On the positive side, nitrites inhibit various bacteria, including botulism, from growing. Nitrites induce several side effects, but their main danger lies in their carcinogenic potential when they are transformed into nitrosamines. This may be especially true for bacon, which, after frying, develops a potential carcinogen, nitrosopyrrolidine. At the current FDA limit of 200 parts per million, no cancer-inducing effect has been seen in experimental animals.

Nitrites have been removed from baby food because of their tendency to combine with hemoglobin (the reaction that, incidentally, causes ham to be pink), converting it to methemoglobin, which, unlike hemoglobin, does not transport oxygen effectively.

Our ability to purchase our food at reasonable prices and to have a vast selection of foods grown and shipped from all over the world, regardless of season, depends on the technology and distribution skills of the food industry. We cannot all grow our own food. To grow, harvest, process, package, and distribute the thousands of food articles of acceptable taste, quality, and safety requires the use of many different pesticides and food additives in order for the products to reach our table. As we have seen in this section, our bounty may not be without mixed blessings.

Obesity

Obesity ranks as one of the leading disorders in this country. It is a disease that is generally insidious in onset, chronic in nature, and very difficult to treat effectively. The overweight patient usually has gained several pounds a year, and over a period of years finds himself many pounds overweight. Most people who are overweight have a strong desire to reduce but lack the willpower and endurance to achieve successful weight reduction. If for a period of ten years or so one gains two or three pounds per year, there may be a 20- to 30-pound excess in weight.

The causes of obesity are complex. Overweight often begins in childhood and continues into adult life. The overweight adult who has had a weight problem from childhood not only has large fat cells (cells that store fat) but a greater number of fat cells than a non-obese person. Even with weight reduction, with fat cells that have shrunk due to loss of depot fat, the obese patient still has more fat cells in his body.

Certainly, psychological factors are most important in obesity. Food is one of our major sources of gratification. This relationship begins when the infant's first contact with the outside world is provided by means of feeding. Our technology, which has made food so available, has also introduced many new forms of frustrations and reduced some satisfactions. We no longer have such close family ties, and our jobs often lack a sense of individual accomplishment or satisfaction. These and many other causes of frustration increase the need for other types of gratification.

Agricultural America has become industrial America. Food is provided for millions who have migrated from rural communities into sprawling urban complexes. No longer do we need to work from dawn to sunset for our daily bread. We rely on others in distant locations and our technology to supply most of our needs. We work our forty-hour week and strive for economic success. Many of us drive great distances to work at a rapid pace, usually in our own cars or by public transportation. We speed on the highways to reach our destination, often caught up in traffic snarls or packed in buses or subways. We rely on elevators instead of stairs and on phones or intercoms to communicate with others. Our bodies are spared the physical efforts, but the technology we use so effectively creates many feelings of frustration which often are relieved by a snack or a large meal. There is a regular need to soothe anxieties or combat disappointments built up as we mull over our jobs, various unsatisfactory contacts with people, marital difficulties, inability to communicate effectively with our children, and concerns and anxieties over health and finances. For many persons, food is a means of quenching these feelings.

For the person who derives comfort from eating, food is plentiful and quite inexpensive in relation to other expenditures. Our technology provides for storage of food in freezers and allows for rapid transportation and availability of all varieties of food articles. Processing of foods and ease of storage permits the average homeowner to walk but a few feet and sample all sorts of goodies. With a little more effort, a trip to the local pizza house or to a drive-in for a hamburger is easily accomplished.

It is hard to escape the constant barrage of movies, television programs, and advertising, all of which stress the neat and slim look, which is especially emphasized for women. The person with a weight problem often becomes further depressed because of inability to measure up and may even gain more weight. Rather than cut down on eating, the combination of loss of self-respect and the resulting depression causes him to eat with an even greater compulsion.

Some housewives hate to waste food, having been brought up by parents of the Great Depression era, and must finish all the food that is served. Under the guise of economy, they polish off whatever is left on their children's plates. Husbands may not notice their wives' weight gain, or may not care. The housewife continues to overeat, compensating for a lack of attention, and obesity becomes a regular way of life.

Physicians almost daily hear the same statement from the overweight patient: "I cannot understand my weight problem because I eat less than any of my friends or my family." Yet when such a person is put into a hospital and given a strictly supervised diet with controlled calorie intake, weight loss almost always occurs at the anticipated rate. If one asked an obese housewife who made this claim to record everything she ate, a typical day would begin with her eating cereal, coffee, and buttered toast. She would then finish her son's cereal and eat the remnants of her daughter's toast and bacon. Preparing the evening dinner, she would taste the chicken soup several times in the process of making it, sample the mashed potatoes, and then try the whipped cream frosting for dessert. After dinner she would finish some salad and meat-loaf, and although not cutting herself a piece of cake, would finish off her daughter's dessert. Such patients become obese by sampling everything they cook and finishing up the left-overs on everyone else's plates.

The average overweight patient has made more than one attempt to lose weight. There is no simple program that will reverse the years of overeating and gradual weight gain; on the contrary, a diet will require many weeks and months of dedication to be effective. What starts out as a firm resolution to lose weight often lasts but a few days, and then the obese person capitulates to the ever-existing pressures and tensions by going back to the previous dietary habits. The several days of calorie-watching are quickly dissipated by one night at a fish fry or by eating a piece of pecan pie.

At some point, usually through the efforts of a friend or family member or a physician, the obese patient joins a weight-reducing club. Sensible dieting is discussed and sessions are often productive. The weekly meetings are, in fact, a form of group psychotherapy, and bring people together to discuss and share their problems with weight reduction. This sense of sharing a problem with others and seeking a solution together often produces results over a period of months. In addition, the competitive spirit of achieving the goal set by the group adds to the effectiveness of the program. However, at some point, often after months, either because of the diet restrictions that are required or from a practical desire to save the small fee that is charged, the person may drop out of the program. Three months and perhaps 25 or 30 pounds later, with the willpower no longer reinforced by supportive group sessions, the reformed dieter returns to his former eating habits and regains all the lost weight in a matter of several weeks and, in fact, often rebounds to a greater weight than before the program. Once the group's positive influence for weight reduction has been eliminated, a second helping of dinner or a piece of cake once again soothes the dieter's pressures and anxieties.

Every obese patient should consult with his physician for an evaluation and a discussion of his problem. A thorough physical examination should be done to rule out the small possibility that the weight problem is, in fact, a symptom of a glandular disorder, namely, an underactive thyroid gland or hypothyroidism. Unfortunately, most overweight patients have normal metabolisms and thyroid function and are not victims of an underactive thyroid gland. The visit with the physician allows a discussion of personal problems that may have aggravated their frustrations and prevented effective attempts at weight reduction. An effective and safe diet can be discussed and given as a guide for the patient to follow. Often, a few simple suggestions may prove of major benefit to a particular patient with a weight problem (such as eliminating desserts or alcoholic beverages). A discussion of the value of weight reduction for general good health may also provide the stimulus and motivation for a particular patient.

However, a visit to the physician's office and instruction on weight reduction with a written diet does not guarantee success by any means. Weight reduction occurs only by following the diet and using the period of weight reduction to restructure eating patterns and habits. As weight reduction is begun, other means of coping with anxieties and frustrations must be sought. These include developing meaningful relationships with our friends and loved ones as well as striving to develop ourselves so that satisfaction results from our jobs, avocations, hobbies, community interests, etc.

All too often, the obese person is a victim of his vice and goes from one doctor to another looking for an easy solution. Health spas thrive by catering to the obese. All sorts of fad diets, food substitutes, and mechanical gimmicks are available, offering a solution which, at best is usually only temporary, and often of no value at all. Yet, any glimmer of hope is sought and almost any book may become a best seller if it is devoted to the topic of weight reduction and a new, easy means to achieve it.

Physicians are usually asked for pills and drugs for weight reduction, but most are reluctant to use medicines for this goal. Weight loss may occur, but generally obesity is not reversed. Diuretics or fluid pills will cause a weight loss in all people, including the thin and non-obese. These drugs work on the kidneys and cause the loss of salt and water. Their effects are temporary and the weight—salt and water—quickly returns. Their long-term use can cause serious side-effects, including a loss of the important mineral potassium.

Amphetamines are a class of drugs that have been used effectively as appetite suppressants. However, appetite-suppressant drugs are addicting, have many side-effects (including over-stimulation followed by depression), and are potentially harmful to patients who may have undiagnosed heart disease. Their use should be generally discouraged and offered only as a temporary measure for a particular individual who may need special help to initiate a diet program.

The use of thyroid hormone is indicated for the probably less than 5 percent of patients who are overweight and found to have thyroid disease. The use of pills for combatting obesity only treats the symptoms of a deep problem and does not force the person to face the problem of learning to channel needs for gratification and develop self-assurance and self-esteem.

Weight reduction can be achieved. Our body processes require fuel or energy to function properly. Our energy needs are expressed by a unit called a calorie. Weight gain occurs when we consume daily more calories than our body expends performing our activities. Weight loss occurs only when our activity level requires more calories than are provided by our food. When more calories are required to make up for the deficit provided in our diet, the body uses and relies on our body reserves or fat depots that are stored in our fat cells, and weight loss occurs.

Sticking to a diet that gives the patient fewer calories than are needed will result in weight reduction. Common sense in selecting the proper food also goes a long way toward maintaining a proper calorie intake. An apple is less fattening than a piece of pie, but eating several apples is equivalent to eating a piece of pie. If an apple furnishes 75 calories, or energy units, and a piece of pie 300 calories, eating four apples is equivalent to eating a piece of pie. Therefore, dieting involves selecting foods that have fewer calories and are, therefore, less fattening, as well as eating a reasonable portion of food. Everyone knows overweight people who throw up their hands claiming they cannot lose weight despite avoiding pastries, starches, etc., and nibbling in between meals. They claim that they eat only a salad and a piece of steak. But how big a steak! Once again the dieter must select the right food and eat only a reasonable portion in order to reduce the intake of calories.

Obviously, a laborer will require a different calorie level than an inactive middle-aged person. An obese patient should discuss with his physician his desire for weight reduction and follow a diet recommended by him based on calories that can be eaten daily. The first patient may lose weight on a 1,500 calorie diet, the latter on a 1,000 calorie diet. Once a given diet is selected, all foods may be eaten, provided the total number of calories is not exceeded. Generally, however, the fattening type of foods—potatoes, fried foods, pastries, breads, sweets, etc.—are avoided because their calorie values are high and they do not leave enough calories for other important and satisfying foods.

As stated earlier, an overweight patient must be committed to follow a diet for a long period of time. Several days of adhering to a diet achieves no results if one "cheats" frequently. Also, one must not be discouraged by day-to-day performance. Rather, the obese person should chart his weight weekly so that the slow weight loss becomes more meaningful and psychologically beneficial.

In dieting there is no need to buy special and more costly diet foods, but, generally, diet beverages may be quite useful. However, all diet beverages are not necessarily low in calories. Since the cyclamate scare, saccharin has been widely used again as an artificial sweetener, so that sugar may be added to improve the taste. So, one must read the label and note the number of calories in each ounce.

Exercise alone does not generally produce significant weight reduction. Here, too, perspiration produces salt and water loss, which is restored when we drink or eat. Again, weight reduction occurs only when our expenditure of calories exceeds our intake of calories. The average person who is not a professional athlete is unable to increase his exercise effort sufficiently to lead to weight loss unless the exercise is accompanied by decreased intake of calories. Exercise is beneficial for several other reasons. Psychologically, exercise, especially if pleasurable (bowling, tennis, swimming) produces gratification and satisfaction, the lack of which often leads to compulsive eating. Furthermore, it removes us from our homes and keeps us away from snacks, thus reducing the opportunity for calorie consumption. Also, the effort of regular exercise, perhaps getting up one hour earlier in the morning to jog, reinforces our motivation later in the day to resist the temptation to eat more food. Exercise also tends to improve muscle tone, making us feel and look better, which, again, provides an additional stimulus to follow a diet.

Often a serious dieter does succeed in achieving substantial weight loss. If his clothes are then quite large, the old clothes should be discarded or altered so they won't be available in the back of the closet for reuse if weight gain recurs. The cost of new clothes is a constant reminder to keep the weight down and to watch calories. Once a satisfactory weight level has been achieved, dieting or watching what we consume has to be a regular activity. Often after the desired weight is achieved, continued dieting is necessary Monday through Friday, let's say, so that the usual overindulgence that occurs on weekends does not cause a return to the former weight level. A few pounds gained over the weekend can be trimmed by watching the diet during the week.

Finally, weight loss is a slow process and the obese person should not get discouraged provided weight loss is occurring. Our fat depots are a rich supply of body energy, and a little goes a long way in running our body machinery. The body stores of fat provide a rich source of fuel to the obese person who is on a diet, so that they are depleted slowly, but even one pound of weight loss per week adds up to a significant reduction over several months' time.

Smoking

The disapproval of tobacco in any form, for smoking, chewing, or snuff, goes back many centuries. The objections to tobacco smoking, in cigars, pipes, or cigarettes, include social ones as well as known and suspected health hazards. To the nonsmoker, having to breathe air contaminated by tobacco smoke is unpleasant. Horace Greeley described a cigar as "a fire at one side and a fool at the other."

Efforts to limit smoking have included penalties and punishments. The English King James I, in 1604, tried to use the power of the monarchy when he declared smoking "barbarous, beastly, hateful to the nose, a vile and stinking custom, harmful to the brains, dangerous to the lungs."

In Turkey, anyone caught smoking a pipe had his nose pierced with it; but despite this punishment, the habit persisted, and in 1633 the Sultan imposed the death penalty for smoking. A similar fate awaited anyone caught selling tobacco in China, and in Russia, the penalty was exile to Siberia. Smoking in public was prohibited in Germany until 1848, and smoking in church was reason for excommunication in the 17th century.

More recently, efforts to limit and discourage cigarette smoking, because of its health hazards, have focused on public education, prohibition of cigarette advertising from television, and the direct warning which appears on all cigarette packages, "Warning: The Surgeon General Has Determined That Cigarette Smoking Is Dangerous to Your Health." Despite past and present attempts to curtail tobacco use, smoking has continued to flourish and tobacco use has increased.

People continue to smoke cigarettes despite convincing statistics which show that cigarette smokers have shorter lives than nonsmokers and that heavy smokers die sooner than light smokers.

Cigarette smoking is associated in various degrees with several important causes of death, including cancer of the lung, chronic bronchitis and emphysema, and coronary artery disease.

The evidence linking lung cancer and cigarette smoking has been substantiated in several studies, including the *Report of the Advisory Committee to the Surgeon General of the United States Public Health Service* (1964)—*Smoking and Health*.

In a British study, those who smoked more than 25 cigarettes a day had a death rate 30 times that of nonsmokers for cancer of the lung, and those smoking less still had 13 times the death rate compared to nonsmokers.

In addition, other types of upper respiratory cancers—cancers of the mouth and larynx as well as of the esophagus—have a higher incidence in smokers compared to nonsmokers.

Cigarette smoking is strongly linked to chronic bronchitis. Many studies have shown that smoking produces changes in the cells lining the airways of the lung and also impedes the normal cleansing mechanism of the bronchial tubes.

Other studies show smokers have more frequent upper respiratory infections, such as colds, which last longer and cause greater absenteeism from work compared to those of nonsmokers.

Statistical data support the increased risk of coronary artery disease among smokers versus nonsmokers. An ongoing study from Framingham, Massachusetts, shows heart attacks occur 2.4 times more frequently among cigarette smokers.

Many other possible associations between cigarette smoking and health problems have been raised but are less definite. Ulcer disease, and even skin wrinkling have been linked to cigarette use. Pipe and cigar smokers who do not generally inhale their tobacco directly, other than from the increased concentration present in the air around them, do not show the increased risk cigarette smokers have for lung cancer, chronic bronchitis, or coronary artery disease.

One reason for continued efforts to get people to stop their smoking habit is that the risk of developing cancer of the lung falls substantially once they no longer smoke. After 10 years of nonsmoking, a former smoker has the same risk of developing lung cancer as one who had never smoked.

The rights of nonsmokers are being recognized more and more. Areas where smoking is allowed are designated on buses and planes to protect the right of those who object to cigarette smoking or are made ill from cigarette smoke, and some states have passed laws against smoking in stores.

If statistics are not convincing, the attitude of physicians themselves must merit consideration in assessing the dangers of smoking cigarettes. Very few physicians smoke cigarettes. At large medical meetings, with hundreds of physicians in attendance, no one seems to be smoking. There has to be good evidence behind it to get us to practice part of our gospel— *stop smoking, any way you can.*

Exercise and Fitness

A person who is free of disease certainly is in good health, but it is possible to improve upon this situation. Being physically fit implies more than just a lack of abnormality. The really fit person approaches the ideal in physical stamina and mental alertness. Such a state is attainable by practically everyone by the proper type and the right amount of exercise.

Lack of the right sort of physical exercise causes some of the most common complaints the doctor sees in his practice. The victim of the "tired housewife syndrome" who is "tired all the time," and the "exhausted" middle-aged man who falls asleep shortly after supper every evening in front of the television set are examples of people whose health is not optimal. They are usually found to be free of any detectable disease or abnormality. When the doctor suggests that they exercise more, they quickly protest that they work hard all day. Though they obviously consider their daily fatigue-producing chores to be exercise, this is not the right sort of exercise to attain and maintain fitness.

When many people think of exercise, they think of push-ups and sit-ups, or of weight-lifting, or sometimes of isometrics. These kinds of exercises, however, do not help in developing fitness in the sense we are talking about now. They do help develop specific muscles, and they can be used to increase strength or add bulk to the physique. But to obtain the health benefits we will mention below, you must pursue *aerobic* exercises, or what athletic coaches used to call "wind exercises."

Aerobic exercises are those that require repetitive activity of large muscles, continued long enough to raise the pulse rate significantly and maintain this elevated pulse rate. Examples are brisk walking, jogging, running, skipping rope, swimming, bicycling, and playing handball or tennis.

Many health benefits come from fitness that results from adequate exercise. The amount of air that the lungs can handle is increased, and the lungs process the inhaled oxygen more effectively. Heart function is improved, so that more blood is pumped with each stroke; this enables more work to be done with fewer heartbeats, that is, with a slower pulse. There is a slight drop in blood pressure. The blood vessels increase in number and size, including the coronary arteries. Muscle tone improves. The amount of fat tissue is decreased.

The maximum oxygen consumption is elevated. This is the best objective index of physical fitness, but it requires the equipment of a sophisticated physiological laboratory and so is not available for everyday use. The highest levels are seen in Olympic distance runners.

In addition, the fit person feels better. He is less tense but more wide awake. The knowledge of his or her self-discipline contributes to the increased sense of well-being present in persons who exercise properly.

Almost everyone can exercise, but there are a few medical conditions that might make it dangerous, including certain forms and stages of heart or lung disease, arthritis, and infections. Persons over 30 who haven't been doing some form of exercise, and everyone over 40 years of age, should consult their doctors before beginning an exercise program. An electrocardiogram, and frequently a stress test electrocardiographic study, will often be desirable to help decide how much exercise is good for you.

It is simple common sense to start exercising slowly, and to work up gradually to a desirable level. When exercise is stopped for more than a few days because of illness or any other reason, you should start at a lower level of activity than when you left off, and increase it slowly again.

Jogging has become the classic form of aerobic exercise, and is one doctors frequently recommend. It can be done almost anywhere, at almost any time, alone or in a group, and without any special equipment. Here are some hints on how best to go about it.

Technique. How you jog isn't really important. "Doin' what comes naturally" is as good a way as any. Some pointers may help: (1) Keep your back as straight as is comfortable, and your head up. (2) Breathe with your mouth open. (3) Let your arms swing freely; don't think about them. (4) Your foot should strike the ground with the heel, then roll forward and take off with the ball of the foot. Some joggers do it flat-footed. Don't jog like a sprinter with the ball of the foot and toes providing the initial or only contact with the ground.

Schedule. Jog regularly, either every day or every second day, for 15 to 30 minutes. Start slowly; run 50 to 100 yard segments very slowly, then walk an equal distance. You can gradually increase the distance you run, and later pick up the speed at which you run. When you get to doing a mile in under eight minutes, you're getting too competitive; ten minutes is a reasonable goal, but twelve is acceptable. Don't be intimidated by schedules in books or articles. Work out your own rate of progress, remembering you're in a lifetime program and there's no hurry to achieve any goal.

Where. The ideal course would be easily accessible, level, and soft underfoot; it would have distances marked off, provide interesting scenery, and not be used for other traffic. Places which have some of these qualities are cinder running tracks (often at schools), grassy parks, little-used streets and roads, or even city sidewalks.

To evaluate what you're doing, the course must be measured. An automobile or bicycle odometer is probably the best way to mark your path. A pedometer is satisfactory. Simply counting strides for a 100-yard trip (any football field, goal to goal) and applying this to your jogging track will accomplish the same thing.

When. Some persons prefer the early morning, mostly because once the day is started there doesn't seem to be time. The fringe benefits are fewer spectators, coolness in summer, the feeling of starting the day brighter, and the economy in time, since you'll shower and dress anyway. Noon jogging breaks up the day nicely. Jogging before dinner can unwind you as well as a cocktail. Jogging later in the evening, where practical, is a good ending to the day.

Dress. Any old clothes are fine for jogging. A sweatsuit can be bought at any sporting goods store. In the summer, shorts are best. In the winter, you can wear pants and a jacket over the sweatsuit.

Footwear is the most important item. The ability to absorb shock at both the heel and the ball of the foot is the essential quality for jogging shoes. A good pair of thick-soled sneakers is quite satisfactory. Sweat socks make them more comfortable.

Similar principles apply to other forms of exercise. If you're going to walk, work up to a mile in 15 minutes or less, since desultory ambling isn't very helpful. Whatever you do, sustain the exercise for at least 15 minutes and do it at least three times a week. Gradual warm-up for a few minutes is desirable, and you should allow time afterward to cool down. The Royal Canadian Air Force Exercise Plans are satisfactory, as are the schedules in "The New Aerobics," by Kenneth Cooper.

The Periodic Health Examination

American children and middle-aged executives of large companies have one thing in common: they are the only large segments of our population that generally receive adequate preventive medical attention. This situation is improving, as more and more people are becoming aware of the desirability of health maintenance care. Such care is available at your personal physician's office.

Young adult men who are in good health should have thorough examinations every two or three years. If the initial examination fails to show any health problem, every three years is satisfactory up to the early thirties, and then every two years up to age forty. After forty, an annual examination is desirable. Healthy young women, however, should see their doctor once every year, for at least a blood count, breast examination, and pelvic examination with Pap smears to detect early cancer of the cervix. The reasons for this are that menstruating women have a significant incidence of anemia, that certain forms of cancer can occur in young women, and that the Pap smear is an effective means of detecting very early cancer of the cervix of the womb.

There are two main objectives in having an annual complete checkup after the age of forty. The first is the early detection of disease, which is often possible even in persons who feel perfectly well. Diabetes mellitus and high blood pressure are probably the two commonest conditions the doctor finds in middle-aged persons who consider themselves to be in excellent health. Occasionally an early, unsuspected, curable cancer is found, and it is not rare to diagnose a pre-malignant condition, that is, something which would lead to cancer if not properly treated.

The second objective of the annual health examination is to educate patients in healthful living, specifically in regard to the factors or trends the family doctor sees in these checkups. A few pounds gained each year may be the beginning of obesity, unnoticed unless the doctor brings it to attention. Increasing alcohol use, or excessive smoking, or lack of physical exercise indicate habits which could cause considerable future trouble unless corrective action is taken promptly.

At the first of these periodic health examinations, a detailed medical history is obtained. The person's past history of operations and illnesses is reviewed. His or her family medical history is obtained, in order to be alert to hereditary diseases, or to trends of disease patterns that may be prominent in the family. The history of any allergies, including known drug sensitivity, is important. The doctor will try to get an idea of the person's background and daily life, his or her occupational history, how he or she is adjusting in his or her marriage or in the single state, and in general what his or her daily problems are. The doctor will ask many questions in what he calls a "review of systems." He inquires about symptoms related to each of the body's systems. For example, to determine whether there are any complaints concerning the respiratory system, he will ask about cough, shortness of breath, and chest pain.

The medical history will be much shorter on subsequent examinations. Although the review of systems is unchanged, the doctor needs only to be brought up to date on the remainder of the history.

The *physical examination* requires removal of all your clothes, and the donning of an examination gown. These come in various kinds, none of which would win any fashion prizes. All are large, loose-fitting, and simple.

The examination will include determining your height, weight, pulse rate, and blood pressure, some or all of which will be done by the nurse. The doctor examines the pupils of your eyes and your eye movements, and using a special light called the ophthalmoscope, inspects the optic disc and the blood vessels in the retinas of your eyes. The ears, tongue, and throat are looked at. He then feels for lymph nodes in your neck, the carotid pulses, and the thyroid gland in the front of your neck. He listens to your breathing and to your heartbeat in several areas of the chest. The breasts are carefully examined. He feels your abdomen to look for masses, or enlargement of the liver, spleen, and kidneys. The groins are examined for lymph nodes and the femoral pulses. The reflexes in the extremities are checked, including scratching the sole of the foot, which tells the doctor more about the brain and spinal cord than about the feet. The pulses at the ankle and foot are important in telling about the circulation. The last parts of the examination in a man will be checking for hernia, and the rectal examination. The latter tells about the prostate gland as well as the rectum itself. Any stool (feces) on the examination glove can be tested for the presence of blood at that time. In a woman, in addition to a rectal exam, a vaginal examination allows assessment of her pelvic organs including the ovaries and uterus, and a Pap smear is obtained. This is sent to a cytology laboratory for staining and inspection for pre-malignant or malignant cells. The skin is observed during the course of the general examination, and any abnormalities are noted. The movement and appearance of the major joints are examined briefly during the examination of the extremities.

Frequently a proctosigmoidoscopic examination will be done—"procto" for short. This involves inspection of the lowest ten inches of the rectum and colon through a hollow tube with a light system. To do this adequately an enema is almost always necessary to prepare the bowel. When done as a diagnostic procedure, this is not a painful experience, although there may be an uncomfortable urge to have a bowel movement. The presence of anal disease such as an acute thrombosed hemorrhoid does make this exam painful. A special table is used for this procedure which allows for the necessary position: head down, anus up. Five percent of men over forty years old have one or more rectal polyps, a premalignant condition, in the eyes of most doctors, which is best diagnosed by this sort of examination. Hemorrhoids, colitis, and other anal disease may also be found with this exam, but most important of all, many cancers of the colon (the second commonest cancer in men) are accessible to this examination.

Laboratory tests are part of the periodic health examination. Blood is obtained by means of a venipuncture, that is, a needle inserted almost painlessly under the skin and into the vein for the drawing off of a small amount of blood. The amount needed may seem enormous to the person from whose body it is being taken, but actually only tiny amounts are withdrawn. A complete blood count and urinalysis are always done, as well as blood chemical tests. These last include tests for blood sugar and cholesterol and triglycerides (the fats in the blood). Usually a battery of twelve tests is done all at once in a special "sequential analyzer," which gives a "profile" of liver and kidney functions, serum calcium, blood proteins, uric acid, and one or more enzymes.

A chest x-ray is part of the initial checkup, but probably won't be necessary every year except for heavy smokers (20 or more cigarettes a day) or persons who have other special risks for lung or heart disease. Other x-rays may be done depending on the history and physical findings. In general, x-ray studies are not routine, but rather done for specific indications. Mammography, x-rays of the breasts, may detect early breast cancer before the tumor can be felt. X-rays are completely painless, and most resemble having a photograph taken. X-rays in this day and age are also safe, because modern equipment allows for thorough examination with the most minimal x-ray exposure.

A baseline electrocardiogram is useful and should be

repeated periodically. Even if perfectly normal this has value as a basis for comparison in the future during a study of obscure chest pain. The electrocardiogram, like the chest x-ray, is completely painless. Small metal electrodes are attached to the four extremities, and a movable electrode is placed on various areas of the chest during different parts of the electrocardiogram. The electrical activity given off with each beat of the heart is recorded on a continuously moving strip of paper. Interpretation of this graph requires training and experience which not all doctors have.

Occasionally a "stress electrocardiogram" is done on a periodic health examination; this involves maximum exercise on a stationary bicycle or a treadmill. It is a very accurate means of finding coronary artery disease. However, it is a time-consuming process which is quite expensive, and is usually done only in special circumstances when heart disease is suspected.

An integral part of the periodic health examination is the *conference* with the doctor to discuss the results. It is at this time that the health education function is carried out, and any abnormalities found can be discussed. Treatment is then prescribed if necessary. At this conference patients should ask questions, and frequently many concerns about which the doctor is unaware can be brought up. Since patients often worry about things that are either unimportant or even normal, doctors welcome the opportunity to offer reassurance about such findings.

When arranged in advance, the entire checkup can be done in two visits, an initial one, which takes from one to three hours, and the later one for the conference on the findings, which usually takes about ten to fifteen minutes. Where special studies are necessary, such as special x-rays, an additional visit may be involved. The cost of the periodic health examination varies, especially depending on what laboratory or other tests are done, but should be between $60 and $150. This is a small price to pay once a year for the knowledge that your health is good, or for the early diagnosis of treatable disease.

DISEASES OF THE HEART AND BLOOD VESSELS

2

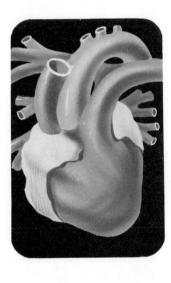

The Circulatory System and Heart

The cell is the basic building block of every form of life. Every free-living plant and animal is made up of one or more cells. Some animals, like the ameba, have only one cell and are so small that they can be seen only with a microscope. The single cell carries out all the life functions. An ameba must live in a watery medium, such as a pond, or the liquid intestinal contents of a larger animal. Its nutrients drift up to the outer lining of the ameba, called the cell membrane, and are engulfed into the interior of the cell, where they are used in the metabolism, or chemical reactions, of the tiny animal. Waste products are excreted through the cell membrane into the surrounding fluid.

A human being is made up of billions of cells, each of which must also receive nutrients and oxygen for its own chemical processes, and its waste products must be taken away. Each of these cells has a surrounding watery medium which bathes the cell, making life possible. This interstitial fluid is minute in amount, and so must continually be renewed. The fluid derives from the blood and it is transported in the circulatory system.

The circulatory system exists solely for the transport of

blood. The many functions of the blood are discussed in Chapter 11. Here we are interested in how the blood is delivered to and from every cell in the body. The heart is a pump that propels the blood through a system of elastic tubes, called *arteries*, to all parts of the body. The arteries branch and decrease in size as they lead to each small area of supply, much like branches of a tree, so that a twig (arteriole) brings blood to all the parts of every organ. (See illustration 1.) By this time the pulsing nature of the flow is converted to a steady gentle current. In other words, as the heart beats a rush of blood flows into the large arteries, and this occurs once a second or perhaps a little faster; the rush is damped by the elastic walls of the arteries, and finally at the end branches, the pressure has been lessened but the flow is smoother. The blood is brought back to the heart to be pumped out again by a thinner, less rigid set of tubes called *veins*. (See illustration 2.) Tiny venules leave the area supplied by an arteriole and usually run alongside the arterial tubes, coming together and getting larger but fewer as they get closer to the heart.

If the heart pumps blood through the arteries to all the organs, and the veins bring it back to the heart to complete the cycle and be pumped out again, then how do the oxygen and nutrients get to the fluid surrounding the cell and how do the cells' waste products get back into the blood? This was a major puzzle that could not be solved until the invention of the microscope, which enabled us to look at the tiny fine details of all the organs and tissues of the body. It was found that the arterioles branch into even smaller tubes whose wall is only one cell thick. (Yes, even the tubes are made up of cells. When you get to these tiny tubes the cells of its wall are flat sheets rolled to form hollow cylinders). These, the smallest of all blood vessels, are called *capillaries*. There are literally billions of capillaries in the human body. Their walls are so thin that the fluid part of the blood contained in the capillaries can flow in and out of these tubes, so that it is in direct contact with the interstitial fluid bathing each cell. Oxygen, molecules of minerals, foodstuffs, and hormones, etc., in the blood diffuse out across the capillary wall, and the carbon dioxide and other molecules excreted by cells into the interstitial fluid diffuse in across the capillary wall and become part of the blood. Although each is small, there are so many capillaries in our bodies that an average adult has a total surface of 68,000 square feet of capillary walls! Obviously

The Major Arteries of the Body

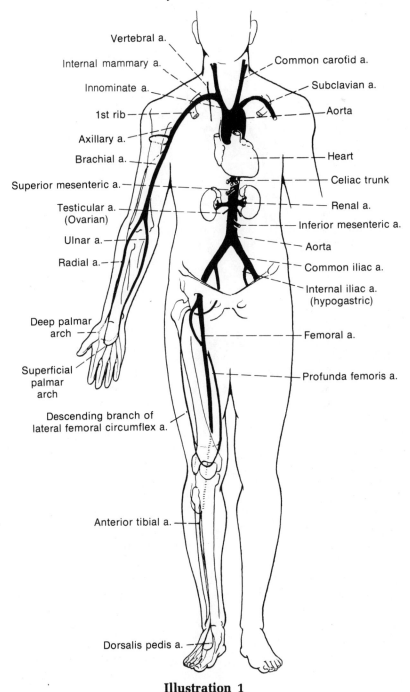

Vertebral a.

Internal mammary a.

Common carofid a.

Innominate a.

Subclavian a.

1st rib

Aorta

Axillary a.

Brachial a.

Heart

Superior mesenteric a.

Celiac trunk

Testicular a.
(Ovarian)

Renal a.

Inferior mesenteric a.

Ulnar a.

Aorta

Radial a.

Common iliac a.

Internal iliac a.
(hypogastric)

Deep palmar
arch

Femoral a.

Superficial
palmar
arch

Profunda femoris a.

Descending branch of
lateral femoral circumflex a.

Anterior tibial a.

Dorsalis pedis a.

Illustration 1

The Major Veins of the Body

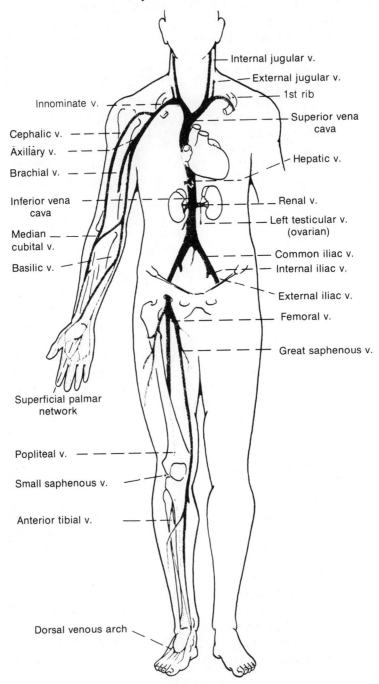

Internal jugular v.

External jugular v.

1st rib

Innominate v.

Superior vena cava

Cephalic v.

Axillary v.

Hepatic v.

Brachial v.

Inferior vena cava

Renal v.

Left testicular v. (ovarian)

Median cubital v.

Basilic v.

Common iliac v.

Internal iliac v.

External iliac v.

Femoral v.

Great saphenous v.

Superficial palmar network

Popliteal v.

Small saphenous v.

Anterior tibial v.

Dorsal venous arch

Illustration 2

exchange by diffusion in and out of the interstitial fluid is made easier by this large amount of filtering area. Capillaries drain into the *venules,* so that there is a continuous circuit of tubes of various sizes through which the blood flows.

Let us now look at the pump that keeps the blood moving through the circulatory system. In a normal adult, the heart weighs between one-half and three-quarters of a pound. It consists of four chambers: a right atrium, a right ventricle, a left atrium, and a left ventricle. (See illustration 3.)

Blood returning from the organs and tissues empties finally into two large veins, the superior vena cava from the head and neck structures and the upper extremities, and the inferior vena cava from the rest of the body. The two vena cavas drain into the right atrium, and then through the tricuspid valve into the right ventricle. When the muscle that makes up the wall of the right ventricle contracts, the tricuspid valve shuts, and the blood in the ventricle is pushed out through the open pulmonic valve into the main pulmonary artery, and then to the lungs.

In the lungs, oxygen is added to the blood, and it returns via the pulmonary veins to the left atrium. The blood traverses the mitral valve into the left ventricle. The wall of the left ventricle is the thickest part of the heart, because its muscle is required to do the most work. When the left ventricle contracts, the mitral valve shuts so that there is no back-flow into the left atrium, and the aortic valve opens. The blood is then propelled out of the left ventricle into the aorta, the largest artery in the body, from which all the other arteries ultimately branch.

The two ventricles contract together. Blood is pumped into the lungs at the same rate that blood is pumped out to the rest of the body. When the body is at rest, the heart beats between 60 and 100 times per minute, although in some people it may be a little slower. With exercise, the heart rate increases, because the tissues need more oxygen. At an average rate of 72 per minute, just think how often your heart beats in a year, or in a lifetime!

Cardiovascular Disease—A Survey

Over half of all deaths in the United States are due to disease of the heart and blood vessels, representing a toll of well over a million lives annually, or three times as many deaths as are caused by cancer. More than 27 million Americans were esti-

Circulation in the Heart

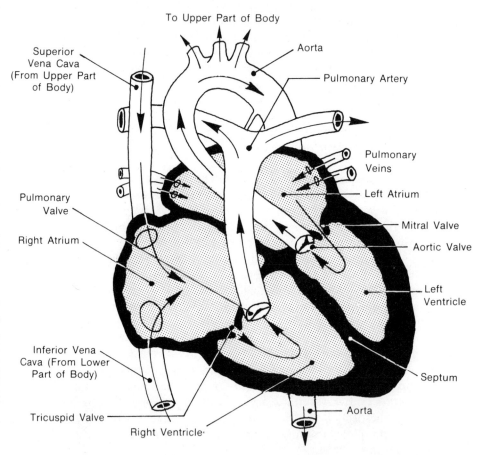

The right side of the heart receives oxygen-poor blood which is pumped to the lungs through the pulmonary arteries. The left side of the heart receives blood from the lungs which is enriched with oxygen and delivers it throughout the body.

Illustration 3

mated to have suffered some form of cardiovascular disease in 1974. The American Heart Association tells us that the cost of cardiovascular disease in 1974 was $19.7 billion.

By far the commonest of all the many diseases of the circulatory system is high blood pressure. Its importance lies in the fact that elevated arterial pressure is one of the causes of atherosclerosis, which produces narrowing of the involved arteries. When the arteries nourishing the heart muscle are affected, the resulting heart disease is the commonest cause of cardiovascular deaths. High blood pressure and atherosclerotic heart disease will be examined in detail in later sections of this chapter.

Next in importance to hypertension and atherosclerosis is rheumatic heart disease, that is, heart disease due to rheumatic fever. The United States Public Health Service has estimated that 1,700,000 Americans have rheumatic heart disease.

Some persons are born with heart disease. Out of every 1,000 births, approximately nine babies have an abnormality of the heart or the large blood vessels arising from the heart. They are said to have *congenital heart disease*. Most of these can be treated successfully, usually with surgery. Only a few of the causes are known. Mothers who develop German measles during the early stages of the pregnancy often have children with heart defects, among other abnormalities. The drug thalidomide, when used in early pregnancy, has been associated with several different forms of congenital heart disease. Congenital heart disease may be hereditary, that is, passed on from generation to generation via the genes. Mutation, or change, of a single gene in one parent can also result in congenital heart disease in some cases.

The development of the heart in the fetus in the mother's womb is a complicated process, and it is not surprising that things can go wrong. Holes can occur in the septa, or tissues that separate the right and left sides of the heart. Valves may be malformed. A narrowing can occur in the aorta. The large blood vessels can be transposed so they attach to the wrong part of the heart.

When the congenital defect causes a shunt, so that blood that has already circulated to the organs and tissues is diverted into the aorta without receiving a new supply of oxygen, cyanosis occurs. This means that because the blood has less oxygen it has a darker color, and the skin becomes blue or "cyanotic." The so-called blue baby usually has this sort of congenital heart disease. Many times shunts do not occur, or else the shunt throws oxygenated blood into the pulmonary circulation, and the person has serious heart disease, but no cyanosis.

Some forms of congenital heart disease are incompatible with life, and these babies die before anything can be done to help them. On the other hand, some forms of congenital heart disease may not result in signs or symptoms until many years later, and in fact the diagnosis is occasionally made for the first time even in a middle-aged patient.

The heart may be damaged as a result of various infections, injury, tumor growth, metabolic disorders, primary muscle disease, and certain toxins or poisons. Syphilis was once a common cause of heart disease, but now that this disease is curable in the early stages, the incidence has lessened considerably. Overactive thyroid, or hyperthyroidism, is a curable cause of heart disease, but most patients with thyroid disease do not have this complication. In certain persons, alcoholic beverages can cause cardiomyopathy, or damage to the heart, which can be fatal.

Rheumatic Heart Disease

Rheumatic fever follows an infection by a certain sort of Streptococcus germ. The overwhelming majority of persons who are infected by this microorganism develop only sore throat, fever, swollen lymph nodes in the neck, diffuse aches and pains, and a generally sick feeling, and then make a complete recovery. However, about 1 out of 100 victims of "strep" (actually the incidence in different epidemics has varied from 3 in 1,000 to 3 in 100) will develop rheumatic fever. The symptoms may overlap those of the strep infection, or may follow a few weeks later. Sometimes the original strep infection is so mild that it is completely overlooked, and the patient cannot remember any illness preceding the onset of his rheumatic fever. It is not yet known why some persons develop rheumatic fever while most do not, but it is thought that there is an abnormality in the normal body defense to the Streptococcus, and this abnormal reaction of the "immune system" causes the inflammatory changes that characterize rheumatic fever.

Most cases occur in children between the ages of 7 and 14, but it may occur at any age, although it is quite unusual below the age of 2 or after 25. The symptoms of rheumatic fever depend upon the location of the inflammation. Arthritis is the commonest complaint, associated with fever. Rash, abdominal pain, nosebleed, and chorea may occur. This last consists of awkward, uncontrollable movements, clumsiness, and brief facial contortions, and is often called St. Vitus' dance. The most important involvement of rheumatic fever, however, is in the heart.

About half the victims of rheumatic fever have heart involvement. There is an enormous range in the degree of sickness produced, from congestive heart failure, in which the heart cannot maintain adequate blood flow to the tissues, to no symptoms at all. In this latter case, there may be merely a murmur heard by the doctor or an electrocardiographic abnormality to signify that the heart is involved.

After the acute illness has subsided, and the patient seems to have made a complete recovery, he still may have a recurrence if he should contract another strep sore throat. For this reason, doctors prescribe long-term treatment with small doses of penicillin—preventive doses rather than treatment doses. Penicillin is extraordinarily effective in killing the particular Streptococcus that is involved in rheumatic fever. Accurate diagnosis of strep throat is made by means of throat culture, and adequate treatment with penicillin of all cases of strep sore throat is an effective means of preventing rheumatic fever. This explains why this disease has become much less common in the last 30 years.

Even without any detectable recurrence, however, the person who has had rheumatic fever may develop damaged heart valves. This may take many years to cause trouble, and not come to light until long after the attack of rheumatic fever. In fact, many persons with valvular damage due to rheumatic fever do not remember ever having had acute rheumatic fever. It is thought that some cases of the acute disease are so mild that they are shrugged off as a cold, or "growing pains," and no attention paid to what is only a minor discomfort.

Like the original strep sore throat, and the acute rheumatic fever, the damaged heart valves may cause little or no disability. It is not uncommon to discover the condition in an apparently healthy person undergoing a routine health evaluation examination. On the other hand, rheumatic heart disease can cause serious illness and even death. The mitral valve is most often affected. This is the valve between the left atrium and the left ventricle, and when scarring narrows the valve, in a condition called mitral stenosis, blood tends to back up and accumulate in the blood vessels of the lungs. This sort of congestion produces shortness of breath, and occasionally results in coughing up blood. When the valve is damaged so that it does not close properly, mitral regurgitation is said to occur. Under these circumstances the left ventricle has to work harder and becomes enlarged. The aortic valve may undergo similar changes. When the mechanical handicap is severe or long-continued, the heart muscle may not be able to keep up with the extra work load, and heart failure eventually occurs. With aortic stenosis, the coronary arteries do not fill properly, and angina pectoris (described in a later section), fainting, and, rarely, sudden death can occur.

Fortunately, these valvular changes can be corrected by surgery. Mitral stenosis is sometimes relieved by a "closed" heart operation, that is, one in which a mechanical pump is not necessary. Where this is not possible, or where mitral regurgitation or aortic damage is present, the entire valve can be replaced with a plastic valve which does the job very well. Surgery is often not necessary, and medical treatment is usually very helpful.

Infection can occur on a damaged heart valve; this condition is called bacterial endocarditis. Years ago, this was almost always fatal. Since the development of penicillin and other antibiotics, treatment has progressed so that recovery is the rule, although not invariably so.

Coronary Artery Disease

The number one killer of American men is coronary artery disease. Despite the magnitude of this problem, it was only in the early part of this century that doctors first made the diagnosis in living patients. Heart attacks affect more than one million Americans per year. Of the almost 675,000 persons who die of heart attacks each year, 176,000 are less than 65 years of age. The factors that predispose to coronary artery disease appear to be multiple, and include genetic or hereditary factors, dietary factors that influence the level of fats in the blood, tensions of contemporary life, high blood pressure, cigarette smoking, obesity, and lack of regular exercise.

Coronary artery disease occurs because the main blood vessels in the heart become affected by a process known as atherosclerosis, whereby the inner lining of the blood vessel wall undergoes a fatty degeneration and plaque formation.

The exact mechanism by which this process develops is unknown. The net result is that the blood vessel opening or channel becomes narrowed so that less blood is delivered to the muscle of the heart.

Each human heart beats approximately 100,000 times every day. The heart requires fuel, namely oxygen, to perform properly. During periods when the heart undergoes an increased demand, such as in exercise or during anger, the heart muscle requires greater amounts of oxygen. This is somewhat like an automobile motor which needs increased gasoline during acceleration. If the fuel line is clogged, no additional gasoline is brought to the motor and the car sputters; if the coronary artery is narrowed, additional blood flow and oxygen delivery are impeded and angina pectoris, or chest pain, occurs.

Angina Pectoris. Although the typical heart attack may occur without warning, most patients will suffer periodic bouts of angina pectoris. The description of this pain by T. Heberden in the eighteenth century has not been surpassed. The patient with angina quickly learns that the pain is brought on by activity and exertion, and is relieved by rest. The degree of exertion varies from person to person. Some patients are able to do all but the most extreme level of activity without being affected. Others experience the chest pain of angina from even the simplest of actions. Activities that accelerate heartbeat (climbing stairs, raking leaves, sexual relations, anger, etc.) may precipitate an attack of angina. Simply stopping the provoking activity and resting generally relieves the chest pain. Often a medication called nitroglycerine is used to terminate the attacks. The pill is placed under the tongue and dissolves; relief can occur in seconds.

Angina pectoris may follow one of several courses. Some patients may find the attacks gradually decrease in frequency and disappear. The reasons for this improvement are not totally clear, but they possibly include correction of aggravating factors such as obesity or cigarette smoking, or the development of collateral circulation. This last means that new blood vessel channels develop to support areas of heart muscle previously not receiving adequate blood flow.

On the other hand, the patient may continue to experience occasional anginal episodes with excessive activity, but can learn to control the frequency of attacks by slowing his pace and changing his life style. He avoids activities that provoke chest pain. He may continue to be active but allows

greater time for a chore. He may require an occasional nitroglycerine tablet and carries them with him at all times.
Basically he has stable angina pectoris.

Another group of patients have a particularly aggressive
form—crescendo or progressive angina. The patient may have
had stable angina and then developed increasing attacks of
chest pain brought on by small amounts of activity. The attacks may occur even at rest. These patients are in danger of a
heart attack. The attacks may continue despite correction of
risk factors and using various drugs to minimize heart work.
These drugs include long-acting blood vessel dilators and
newer agents that are called beta-blocking drugs. Because the
risk of heart attack is so great in this group of patients, close
physician supervision is mandatory. Evidence of a heart attack
must be sought by monitoring suspicious episodes of chest
pain with an electrocardiogram. Sometimes observation of the
patient for several days in the intensive care unit of a hospital
is necessary to be certain that permanent heart damage has not
occurred.

Myocardial Infarction. Even without crescendo angina
some patients eventually experience a bout of angina that lasts
longer and is not relieved by nitroglycerine, with pain that is
quite severe and that may be crushing in character. Profuse
sweating may occur, and the patient collapses; he may even
die before receiving medical aid. An area of heart muscle has
been deprived of blood flow and oxygen, and the muscle
irreversibly destroyed. A heart attack, or myocardial infarction, has occurred. This usually comes about because of
complete occlusion, or blocking, of a narrowed coronary artery. A blood clot forming on the roughened interior of such a
blood vessel is the usual cause of a coronary occlusion, but
sometimes bleeding in the wall of the artery under a fatty
plaque can do the same thing, and death of heart muscle can
even occur without any sudden changes in the chronically
impaired blood supply.

It is estimated that 50 percent of patients with heart attacks
die at home. Efforts are being made to improve emergency
units especially trained to sustain the victim of a heart attack
until he reaches the full services of a hospital.

The hospital mortality rate has been reduced from about
30 percent to 15 percent by means of intensive care facilities
with improved monitoring devices and newer drugs to control
irregularities of the heartbeat. The greatest number of deaths

occur in the first week of hospitalization, especially in the first 24 to 48 hours.

New techniques are now available to assess whether the coronary artery channels are narrowed. Special x-rays of the coronary arteries can be performed in many medical centers. Almost invariably, significant narrowing of at least one and possibly three coronary arteries can be demonstrated in patients who have had a heart attack. Although this procedure does involve some risk, surgical correction of the narrowed blood vessel may prevent heart attack with its high mortality.

Surgery for Coronary Artery Disease.   Since the late 1960s, an operation to make a bypass of the occluded coronary artery has become an accepted surgical procedure for treatment of some cases of coronary artery disease. This operation consists in the removal of a section of a vein from the leg, which is then sutured from the aorta to the coronary artery, past the point of obstruction. In effect, it provides a new channel for blood to flow through the coronary arteries, directly from the aorta. This new channel bypasses the occluded segment of coronary artery. The operation has been done frequently enough so that it is now relatively safe, with an average mortality rate of about 5 percent. Complications of surgery are possible, but when patients are selected carefully for this form of treatment, it may be quite effective.

Surgery is not indicated in patients with stable angina pectoris. In those who have disabling angina pectoris, so that they are unable to work, the operation may be very beneficial. Its use also seems reasonable where a more serious heart attack is expected to occur in the near future, as in patients with crescendo angina, in those with a certain form of atypical angina which occurs at night, and in disease of the main left coronary artery.

The operation is usually successful in that it relieves the pain of angina pectoris. Recent statistics seem to indicate that it also prolongs life in many patients. Much more information needs to be accumulated, however, before we can definitely say who can best benefit from this sort of treatment. In selected patients, a new technique, using an inflatable tube that is passed through the narrowed area, can open a blocked coronary artery, thus avoiding open-heart surgery.

Causes of Coronary Artery Disease.   Although coronary artery disease is generally considered to be a disorder of middle-aged and elderly patients, the process of atherosclerosis is already advanced in the late teens and twenties in American men. The Korean War provided an opportunity to study blood vessels at autopsy in young American men killed in combat, and surprisingly revealed a high percentage of advanced atherosclerosis in blood vessels. Coronary artery disease can appear in men in their thirties or even younger.

Interestingly, such disease appears less frequently in primitive people. It appears to increase with exposure to the contemporary Western style of living. It has been quite uncommon in Japanese men, but in Japanese-Americans it increases in frequency and approaches the Caucasian incidence. Apparently the exposure to the American way of life and diet pattern increases the predisposition to the disorder. As mentioned above, a genetic predisposition is present in some persons. This should be suspected especially if several relatives have had heart attacks at relatively young ages.

Diabetes mellitus,which is often considered only a disorder of blood sugar, is also a disease of blood vessels with precocious atherosclerosis. Diabetics often have increased blood fat levels, and this provides another explanation for the increase in coronary artery disease.

Patients who have elevated blood fat levels should be treated for this condition by their physician. A long-term study made of many residents of Framingham, Massachusetts, has shown that men with cholesterol levels of more than 260 milligrams per 100 cc. of blood are twice as likely to suffer heart attacks as those with cholesterol levels of 200 milligrams or lower. Weight reduction itself often provides a reduction in the blood level of cholesterol. Avoidance of cholesterol-containing foods often is beneficial, but cholesterol in the blood is largely a product of body metabolism and not of what is eaten. Cholesterol is manufactured by the liver and is needed for the production of many essential body hormones, including the sex hormones. It is estimated that only 20 percent of our blood cholesterol comes from our diet. If avoidance of high cholesterol foods such as egg yolks, animal fats, and dairy products, along with attempts at weight reduction, are unsatisfactory, several types of medications are available to further lower cholesterol. It is more important to control the cholesterol level in a young patient with a family history of coronary artery disease than in an elderly patient who already has advanced atherosclerosis.

Other persons with a strong family history of coronary artery disease may be found by their physicians to have other abnormalities in fat metabolism besides cholesterol. The commonest variety is due to an elevation of a class of fatty proteins—beta lipoprotein—which is caused by excess consumption not of fat, but of carbohydrates or sugars and starches. Therefore this person will not be helped by the low fat or cholesterol diet which is beneficial for reduction of cholesterol levels, but by a reduction of dietary carbohydrates. A high level of a fat-carrying protein in the blood, called high density lipoprotein (HDL), offers some protection against coronary artery disease by carrying cholesterol away from the walls of blood vessels. In the course of a periodic health examination, the physician may order a measurement of blood fat levels, cholesterol and triglycerides, and, if abnormalities exist, he will perform additional tests (lipoprotein electrophoresis) to determine proper dietary management.

Unlike genetic or inherited factors that may predispose to coronary artery disease (and we do not choose our parents), high blood pressure, cigarette smoking, lack of exercise, and obesity are four significant variables that the patient can tackle with the aid of his physician. High blood pressure has been shown by a recent well-controlled Veterans Administration Hospital study to increase the likelihood of a heart attack considerably. Often weight reduction and avoidance of excessive salt in the diet can lower blood pressure levels. The control of high blood pressure requires surveillance by a physician, who may choose to use drugs to lower the blood pressure when it does not respond to the above measures.

Cigarette smokers have an increased incidence of coronary artery disease. Men who smoke more than a package of cigarettes daily run a threefold greater risk of heart attack than those who have never smoked. Smokers have elevated levels of carbon monoxide in their blood, which binds with the red cells and thus competes with oxygen, the fuel needed by the heart muscle.

Exercise is beneficial for the heart. However, it may be a two-edged sword. In middle-aged or older persons, exercise should be undertaken only after a physical examination, including an electrocardiogram. An inactive, middle-aged male who decides to "get into shape" may have been a star athlete in years before, but he cannot attempt the training schedule that was appropriate for his younger years. Exercise after a prolonged period of inactivity must follow a gradually increasing level of activity. Many health clubs and YMCA's have supervised programs specifically designed for a gradual and controlled increase in exercise performance. The principles of exercise are lucidly described by Dr. Kenneth Cooper in his book on aerobics. The purpose of exercise should not be to increase the bulk of muscles generally but to train and condition the heart muscle to beat more effectively. Jogging, swimming, tennis, and bicycling are all beneficial if performed regularly and judiciously. A person may have a pulse at rest of between 80 and 90 beats per minute before beginning a program of exercise. After several months of exercise the heart may now perform effectively at rest at a rate of 60 beats per minute. Twenty beats saved per minute, 1,440 minutes in a day, adds up to a significant reduction and reflects an increased efficiency of our pump—the heart. Regular exercise may also reverse factors that cause atherosclerosis and stimulate the formation of new blood vessels into the heart muscle itself.

The emphasis should be on prevention, on taking the measures that will enhance our chances for survival by altering factors associated with disease processes. Careful attention to diet, regular exercise, avoidance of cigarettes, and periodic health examinations to uncover genetic risk factors and evaluate blood pressure and blood fats, are important.

Blood Pressure

"Blood pressure" is just what it says: the pressure the blood exerts in an artery. We measure it in the brachial artery, the main blood vessel of the arm. A direct measurement can be obtained by inserting a pressure-sensing device inside the artery, but fortunately the blood pressure can be measured indirectly with almost the same degree of accuracy, by a simple instrument called a sphygmomanometer. A cloth cuff containing a distensible rubber bladder is applied to the arm, and the bladder blown up with air, so that it exerts pressure on the arm. Enough air is used so that the pressure it exerts is higher than the pressure inside the brachial artery, and the artery is compressed, shutting off the blood flow in that segment under the cuff. Then the air is slowly released. When the pressure occluding the artery comes down to the level of the pressure inside the artery, then the occluded part begins to open up and the blood starts to flow through again. This can be felt at the wrist where the pulse becomes restored, or else heard with a stethoscope over the brachial artery below the cuff. This level is the systolic blood pressure. What we hear is a thumping noise as the pulsing blood comes through, each thump corresponding to the heartbeat that propels it. As more air is let out of the sphygmomanometer cuff, the thumping stops. This occurs because we have now reached the level of the diastolic blood pressure, where flow is smooth rather than pulsing. The systolic blood pressure is the highest pressure the blood exerts in the artery and the diastolic blood pressure the lowest pressure.

Normal Pressure. What is the normal blood pressure? There is no single number we can give to answer this question. This is because the pressure changes in all of us from time to time, sometimes even from minute to minute, as well as from youth to old age. We read the blood pressure as two figures—the systolic pressure and the diastolic pressure, both expressed as millimeters of mercury. For example, we may say a blood pressure is 120/80 ("one twenty over eighty"). These figures would be high for an infant, normal for an adult, and possibly low for an older person. Most life insurance companies accept 140 or less as a normal systolic pressure and 90 or less as a normal diastolic pressure, without any further question. However, doctors know that the systolic pressure usually increases with age as arteries are less elastic, and the old saw that the systolic blood pressure is "100 plus your age" has some truth to it. The diastolic pressure is less changeable, and under all circumstances a doctor would like it to be less than 100, and preferably 90 or less for an adult.

The systolic blood pressure, and to a much lesser extent the diastolic blood pressure, is elevated by many factors, including emotions, smoking, eating, and exercise. Merely thinking of an attractive member of the opposite sex may cause the systolic pressure to become raised 30 or more millimeters of mercury, say from 140 to 170 or more. Most persons are nervous during a medical examination, and a single blood pressure reading is often falsely high; this is why the doctor has the patient lie down and makes small talk before rechecking the blood pressure. It is an everyday occurrence to see a first reading of 180/96 fall to 140/80 in a few minutes as the patient gets accustomed to the cuff on his arm and is able to relax. The diagnosis of high blood pressure should never be made on a single determination, and is preferably made only when the blood pressure remains elevated on separate days.

Low Pressure. In an otherwise healthy person, low blood pressure is not a health problem and indeed may confer a better than average life expectancy. Low blood pressure, or hypotension, is important only in shock or adrenal insufficiency, or in the uncommon condition "orthostatic hypotension," where the blood pressure drops so much when the patient stands up that he may even faint. Many persons who complain of tiredness have a normal blood pressure of say 96/60, and blame their malaise on low blood pressure when actually a chronic depression or simple lack of exercise is the real cause.

High pressure. High blood pressure, also called hypertension, in contrast to low blood pressure, is an important health problem. In the United States, from 15 percent to 20 percent of the adult population has high blood pressure! Although the condition itself usually doesn't cause any symptoms, if it continues it will result in serious effects on the heart and blood vessels of the brain, the eyes, and the kidneys, with damage to any or all of these organs.

Many persons who have been told they have hypertension will disagree with the statement that the blood pressure elevation itself usually doesn't cause symptoms, because they say that when their blood pressure is up they feel tense and headachy. Actually this is putting the cart before the horse most of the time, and the tension causes the blood pressure to rise, rather than vice versa.

Persons with "labile hypertension," that is, whose blood pressure is high at times and normal at other times, have the best outlook of all hypertensive patients, because heart and blood vessel damage is less frequent and less severe in them than in persons with "fixed hypertension," where the blood pressure is consistently high. Most serious of all is "accelerated hypertension," which is fortunately rare, but which is associated with very high blood pressure levels and rapidly progressing, severe heart and vascular disease, leading to death in a matter of weeks or months unless treatment is instituted and proves to be successful.

Persons who have had labile hypertension for many years frequently later develop fixed hypertension, and about one in twenty-five persons with fixed hypertension will develop accelerated hypertension. In the years since World War II, effective treatment for high blood pressure has become available.

Nowadays almost all cases can be controlled at least to some extent.

Diagnosis. There is much more to the diagnosis than simply taking the blood pressure, because in some patients with hypertension there is a specific cause that can be corrected, with complete cure of the hypertension. First of all, the doctor has to be sure that the patient actually does have high blood pressure. As we have seen above, a single high reading may not mean anything, and it should be repeated several times on different occasions. When it is determined that the person is hypertensive, then special tests are carried out to assess the status of the heart and circulation as well as to determine the cause.

The most important group of causes, both because they are relatively common and because many are curable, is a group of kidney diseases. In fact, almost all of those diseases that cause long-term damage to the kidneys are associated with high blood pressure. It is possible that a person who feels well and who is found to have hypertension on a routine examination may have a kidney problem that requires treatment. There are other unusual causes of high blood pressure that the doctor considers as he sees a new case of hypertension, many of them diagnosable on a general physical examination. Various endocrine diseases, that is, hormone abnormalities, can cause the blood pressure to be elevated, such as some cases of overfunction of the adrenal glands or the pituitary gland.

A dramatic but very rare cause of high blood pressure is a pheochromocytoma, a tumor that secretes hormones that elevate the blood pressure considerably. Coarctation of the aorta is a congenital narrowing of the aorta (the main artery bringing the blood from the heart to the rest of the body) which causes the blood pressure to be high in the arms above the narrowing but low in the legs below the narrowing; it is permanently cured by an operation.

Because of these possible causes of "secondary hypertension" (that is, secondary to something else, such as kidney disease), when a person is found to have high blood pressure he should have further study. A complete medical history and physical examination are mandatory. Special tests include urinalysis and blood cell counts, determination of blood potassium level (for an adrenal cause), urine culture (for kidney infection), blood tests of kidney function, and x-rays of the kidneys. In addition, a chest x-ray and electrocardiogram are necessary, and blood sugar and cholesterol tests are usually desirable.

Usually no specific cause of hypertension is found, and the patient is said to have primary or essential hypertension.

Treatment.   The treatment of essential hypertension, which we will simply call "high blood pressure" from now on, begins with the establishment of a healthful way of living. Exercise, adequate sleep, and regular hours are important, and drug therapy alone without these basic requirements for good health is inadequate. Abnormally stressful life situations, for example, a job with long hours under much pressure or the continuing domestic problem of an abusive alcoholic spouse, are obstacles to the control of high blood pressure. The person with this condition must pursue treatment. He should realize that although he may feel perfectly well at the outset, failure to control his high blood pressure may lead to irreversible damage in the future. Physicians often see persons who have known that they have high blood pressure but who neglect treatment until they have a stroke or a heart attack.

There is no satisfactory dietary treatment for uncomplicated high blood pressure in a person of normal weight. But overweight persons must lose weight, and it often happens that simply dropping to a normal weight will correct a mild or moderate degree of high blood pressure. A weight-reducing diet is absolutely necessary for the obese hypertensive.

Many patients ask whether they should avoid salt (sodium) in their diets to prevent or treat hypertension. In the 1930s, Dr. W. Kempner, of Duke University, found that the complete avoidance of dietary sodium did lower the blood pressure of some patients with severe hypertension. To achieve this and preserve some degree of adequate nutrition, he used a diet almost exclusively of rice, with some fruit for variety. This rice diet was lifesaving for some persons with high blood pressure. Fortunately, a stringent salt-free diet is no longer necessary. Avoiding dietary salt usually does not significantly affect the blood pressure in most cases of mild to moderate uncomplicated hypertension, and furthermore we now have drugs that promote loss of sodium in the urine to achieve the same results as the rice diet. This is true, however, in uncomplicated cases; in some cases of high blood pressure with heart or kidney disease, a low salt diet or salt-free diet is necessary and, in general, people with high blood pressure should avoid excessive amounts of salt in their diet. By this we mean that food may be prepared normally, but no additional salt added at the table, and that heavily salted foods be avoided, such as potato chips and peanuts.

Another common misconception is that hypertensives should avoid exercise. Nothing could be further from the truth. Of course, some persons may have heart or other disease that requires limited activities. But in uncomplicated high blood pressure, exercise is beneficial. See the section on Exercise and Fitness in Chapter 1 for hints on how to proceed.

Drugs for high blood pressure have been developed in recent years, and medication is helpful in almost all hypertensives of more than mild degree.

Mild labile hypertensive patients often respond to a sedative or tranquilizer, such as phenobarbital, Librium, or meprobamate. Reserpine and other extracts of the Indian snakeroot have been used in the past, and have been extremely effective in lowering a mildly elevated blood pressure. These drugs are not as widely used today, because of some cases of depression and other side-effects, especially with high doses. Antihypertensive diuretics are probably the most commonly used agents today, such as chlorthiazide (Diuril) and many similar medications. These are effective, and the mild increase in urine is either not noticed or only mildly annoying. One drawback is that all these diuretics are potentially wasteful of potassium in the urine if their use is long-continued, and potassium deficiency may cause weakness. Other less common side effects are gout in susceptible persons and a mild increase in blood sugar. Generally speaking, however, diuretic drugs are extremely valuable in treating high blood pressure.

Moderate cases may require several drugs. Aldomet (methyldopa) is often the first drug tried and is usually very effective. There is no single effective dose, and the number of tablets taken daily will have to be arrived at by trial and error. Apresoline (hydralazine), Ismelin (guanethidine), Inderal (propranolol), Aldactone (spironolactone), and a host of other drugs are also available to add to the regimen as required. Close supervision is required to arrive at the proper dosage and the proper combination of drugs for each individual. Sometimes the blood pressure drops too quickly, and light-headedness or dizziness may result, especially when the patient first gets out of bed in the morning, when the blood pressure is lowest anyway.

More severe cases may be controlled by the same drugs in larger amounts, or with others known as ganglion blockers, from their mode of action on the nerves that control constricted blood vessels. These drugs accomplish what used to require an operation—bilateral lumbar sympathectomy—in the 1940s and early 1950s. Often hospitalization is desirable to start treatment.

Once a treatment plan appears effective, there is unfortunately no guarantee that it will not need modification in the future. The blood pressure should be checked from time to time, so that changes in drugs and dosage may be made as necessary, and the patient should count on pursuing treatment indefinitely. Trying to stop the drugs when the blood pressure has reached a normal level is almost always futile, because the blood pressure will slowly climb back up.

Cerebrovascular Disease

Cerebrovascular disease, coronary artery disease, and cancer are the three leading causes of death in the United States. (See Appendix 1). Each year cerebrovascular accidents, or strokes, cause approximately 275,000 deaths and disable another 300,000 persons. The cost to society from loss of work and for medical care is estimated to be $7 billion.

Strokes occur because of disease in the blood vessels that bring blood to the brain. The major blood vessels, the internal carotid arteries and the vertebral arteries, one on each side of the neck, give off branches and tributaries that supply and nourish all of the brain. The carotid system travels in the front or anterior portion of the neck and supplies blood to the largest part of the brain. The vertebral system travels in the back of the neck, actually within the vertebral bones, supplying blood to the hind brain (pons and medulla). The two systems actually connect, and are joined by branches on the under surface of the brain in the circle of Willis. The fact that the carotid and vertebral arteries connect provides a margin of safety to adequate blood flow to the brain. If blood flow is prevented in one major vessel, retrograde or backward flow through a connecting tributary may occur and provide needed blood to an otherwise deprived portion of the brain.

The brain is unique in several ways. Unlike most of our body cells, brain cells are unable to reproduce or divide. Our relative brain size and number of brain cells are maximum in childhood. Thereafter, our brain volume decreases and our brain cells degenerate and are not replaced.

The specialized functions of our brain require a constant energy source, which can only be provided by glucose and oxygen in a process called aerobic metabolism. Almost all other body cells, including the heart muscle, can temporarily generate energy without oxygen by an alternate means called anaerobic metabolism.

The brain requires a constant supply of fuel, consuming 150 grams of glucose and 72 liters of oxygen every twenty-four hours. If these substances are not provided even for a period of a few minutes, brain damage occurs. The brain, which weighs about 1,500 grams, receives approximately 20 percent of all the blood pumped from the heart (750 to 1,000 cc. per minute), which provides the needed oxygen and glucose. Each carotid artery receives about 350 cc. and each vertebral artery 100 to 200 cc. of blood per minute.

If effective circulation to the brain or a portion of the brain is not maintained, reversible injury to brain cells (ischemia) occurs, and may progress to cell death (infarction) in minutes. If the heart stops beating, dizziness occurs in six to eight seconds, unconsciousness in thirty seconds, and irreversible brain damage in two to three minutes, leading to death of the brain in five minutes.

Anything that interferes with blood flow or impairs the concentration of oxygen and glucose in the blood can cause injury to brain cells and permanent damage or a stroke. Examples of such include: (1) an overdose of insulin in a diabetic leading to a reduction of the blood sugar, (2) carbon monoxide poisoning causing a reduction of the oxygen content of the blood, (3) an acute reduction in the blood pressure below a critical level such as in shock, (4) polycythemia (thick blood) impairing blood flow in cerebral vessels.

The most common reason for cerebral vascular disease, or stroke, is impaired blood flow to an area of the brain due to cerebral atherosclerosis. In the United States, 70 percent of strokes are due to cerebral thrombosis and the remainder to either intracerebral hemorrhage or emboli, that is, blood clots that originate elsewhere and travel to the brain.

Cerebral Thrombosis, Hemorrhage, and Emboli. Arteriosclerosis may affect all the blood vessels of the body. It is not the aging event, arteriosclerosis, but the formation of atheromatous plaques (the deposition of fatty-like material in the interior lining, or intima, of blood vessels) that causes narrowing and gradual reduction in the opening or channel of blood flow. If the atheromatous plaque forms gradually, even though there is a significant reduction in the channel, no symptoms may develop because of good collateral circulation (blood flow to the area from other blood vessels), as mentioned above.

The same process, atherosclerosis, produces diseases in other areas of the body, depending on the organ involved. When cerebral blood vessels are involved, the brain and its cells may become damaged and a stroke can occur. If the coronary arteries are affected, the heart is vulnerable to angina pectoris, or a heart attack, as described in the previous section. Involvement of the peripheral blood vessels to the legs produces claudication, or leg pain with exercise, and gangrene of the extremity may develop if the circulation to the leg is significantly impaired.

When a stroke develops, some area of the brain becomes permanently damaged or destroyed. Most commonly this event occurs because of a complete occlusion of a blood vessel by an atheromatous plaque (*cerebral thrombosis*) causing death to an area of the brain (*cerebral infarction*).

At times a piece of atheromatous plaque (*embolus*) can break off from a blood vessel and be carried away to lodge in a smaller tributary and produce an occlusion. The embolus can arise from within the heart or from a heart valve and travel into the carotid system. This is especially likely to occur in persons who have an irregular heartbeat from atrial fibrillation, or who have damaged heart valves from rheumatic fever. Persons who have artificial heart valves are also more likely to form an embolus.

Hemorrhage into the brain substance because of rupture of a cerebral blood vessel may also cause a stroke. An aneurysm, caused by a weakened or defective area of a blood vessel wall, may burst, spilling blood into the brain, damaging tissue and causing the brain to swell. Another cause of a stroke is an arteriovenous malformation, which is a birth defect where a high pressure artery flows into a low pressure vein.

Symptoms of a Stroke.   Most persons with advanced cerebrovascular disease do not have symptoms. Stroke generally develops rapidly, reaching a maximum intensity in hours or a few days. Emboli may occur without warning. Hemorrhage may be preceded by a severe headache, although only a tiny fraction of people with headaches have this problem. At times persons with cerebral thrombosis may have some early symptoms that warn of an impending stroke. Since a cerebral thrombosis is due to occlusion of a blood vessel, partial narrowing may lead to transient brain dysfunction which is reversible. These episodes of transient ischemia may occur as recurrent bouts of dizziness, weakness of a limb, numbness of an extremity, mental confusion, and even difficulty speaking appropriately. Generally the episode lasts several minutes to a few hours, and all symptoms regress within 24 hours.

The location of a stroke (that is, the site in the brain) determines the clinical manifestation. The extent of brain damage determines the degree of loss of sensation and muscle weakness or paralysis. Since the blood supply to the brain involves two separate blood vessel systems, the carotid and vertebral, which communicate via connecting blood vessels, the damage to the affected area of the brain may be significantly reduced by good collateral blood flow.

The blood vessel most commonly involved in a stroke is the internal carotid artery or one of its main branches, usually the middle cerebral artery. Involvement of the right carotid artery or middle cerebral artery produces numbness and weakness or paralysis of the left side of the body. Disease in the left carotid system leads to paralysis or numbness in the opposite side of the body. Usually, in a right-handed person, the left side of the brain is the dominant hemisphere and controls speech activity. Complete occlusion of the left internal carotid in a right-handed person may cause paralysis, numbness, and aphasia (inability to speak).

Treatment. The treatment of a stroke victim initially requires efforts to maintain life and support vital functions. Unconscious or comatose persons require measures to maintain an adequate airway for breathing, and suctioning of respiratory secretions is often necessary. Fluids must be given by vein to maintain hydration while avoiding excessive amounts. A catheter is placed in the bladder frequently to allow for passage of urine. Care of the skin and the parts of the body (buttocks, heels, and elbows) that may develop sores due to the long stay in bed is necessary. Good nursing care is especially vital in these patients.

Stroke patients can follow several different courses. Some victims of a stroke lapse into a coma and die. Others make a complete recovery over a period of weeks to months. Most persons occupy an intermediate position, with partial recovery but with some degree of weakness of the affected side persisting. Sometimes this may be a barely detectable weakness of an arm or leg.

Once a stroke patient has recovered from the acute effects of the cerebrovascular accident and is in stable condition, vigorous efforts at rehabilitation are instituted. Initially, exercise may be passive, and involve motion by a therapist to maintain joint function. As soon as possible, the patient is encouraged to attempt sitting and walking and daily exercise to regain strength and function in the involved side. The skills of a physical therapist are important in scheduling and implementing exercises and muscle training. Canes or walkers are helpful in gait training.

Cerebral thrombosis and infarction occur most frequently in persons between 60 and 80, and cerebral hemorrhage is usually seen in slightly younger persons. Predisposing factors for strokes include hypertension, diabetes mellitus, abnormalities in the blood fats, and irregular heartbeats. Vascular disease in other areas is frequent in persons who have strokes.

Identification of persons with these predisposing factors requires periodic health examinations by a physician. Persons with high blood pressure should be seen regularly by their physician and treated in order to reduce the blood pressure. Efforts to control elevated blood lipid levels by appropriate medication and dietary restrictions as well as good control of diabetes mellitus requires physician supervision.

Other Arterial Diseases

In the previous sections on coronary artery disease and cerebrovascular disease, we discovered the importance of atheromatous plaques as factors in reduced blood supply to the heart and brain respectively. The end result of the decreased supply is angina pectoris and myocardial infarction in the case of the heart and stroke when the brain is involved. The same process that reduces blood flow in other arteries produces disease in the organs or tissues nourished by their circulation.

The main artery in the body is the aorta, which arises from the left ventricle of the heart, arches around the chest, giving off important branches to the upper extremities and neck, and then runs downward into the abdomen, where it terminates by dividing into two iliac arteries that supply the circulation to the legs. From its beginning to its end, many important tributaries are given off. Blood from the heart, rich in oxygen, reaches the stomach, liver, small and large bowel, kidneys, and the muscles and tissues of our legs and feet via important channels arising from the aorta.

Peripheral Vascular Disease

Peripheral vascular disease refers to impairment of blood flow to our lower extremities. Although atheromatous plaques tend to develop in the aorta in most people at an early age, they advance to cause significant disease in only a small number of people. Persons with diabetes mellitus are prone to develop advanced peripheral vascular disease at a younger age. When the disease in the aorta is severe enough to cause symptoms in the lower extremities, it occurs in the terminal portions of the aorta.

The narrowed blood vessel is often the iliac artery or its extensions into the leg. The reduction of the opening in the blood vessels may be partial or complete. The severity of symptoms depends upon the extent of narrowing, the condition of the blood vessels further down from the diseased one, and the extent of collateral circulation (blood bypassing the blocked segment through accessory channels). The most common symptoms associated with peripheral vascular disease are leg cramps, especially during activity.

When we walk for a long distance or at a rapid pace, our powerful leg muscles respond to the demand, but they require an increase in fuel, oxygen, to provide the additional energy output. A narrowed blood vessel is unable to increase the blood flow to the muscles, and pain or an ache develops because of a build-up of waste products that cannot be metabolized. If this person slows down or stops, blood delivery once again becomes adequate and the pain gradually subsides. This type of pain is called claudication and is analogous to heart pain or angina pectoris. Depending on the location of the blocked or narrowed blood vessel, the pain may be located in the calf muscles, thigh muscles, or buttocks. A blockage in the aorta itself may be associated with pain in the buttocks and impotence in the male because of an inadequate blood supply to the artery of the penis. The farther away from the heart the disease is in the circulation, the farther down the leg the symptoms develop.

The disease commonly involves the blood vessels of both

legs, but symptoms may only be present in one leg because of more disease on that side or better collateral circulation in the other leg.

In time, the symptoms may worsen, and the patient notices claudication while walking shorter distances even though he slows his gait. In some persons the symptoms remain stable for long periods of time. Not uncommonly a patient has both angina pectoris and claudication. The angina pectoris may be improved because the claudication in the leg forces the patient to stop and rest before chest pain develops.

Peripheral vascular disease may be limited to one area of a blood vessel or be generalized, involving several blood vessels, including smaller branches. In this case, circulatory changes develop in the skin and the tissues farther downstream, namely, the toes and feet. (Both extremities may be involved.) Inadequate nutrition of the skin of the toes and feet is the result. Hair is lost from the toes, the nails are thickened, and the skin is fine and noticeably cooler, especially in the lower leg and foot. The foot becomes pale when elevated and there is a delay in the return of blood when it is lowered. The toes may appear dusky and purplish. At an advanced stage, the tissues of the skin break down and undergo cell necrosis, or death, a situation known as gangrene.

The doctor generally has no difficulty in diagnosing peripheral vascular disease. The symptoms of claudication are straightforward. On physical examination, the physician checks, besides the changes mentioned above, the femoral pulses in the groin, the popliteal arteries located behind the knees, and the two pulses located on each foot. He observes the amplitude of pulsation of these vessels, comparing each side to the other and noting any absence or discrepancy.

The treatment of peripheral vascular disease is based on a careful evaluation of the symptoms and physical findings. Stable symptoms of claudication which can be controlled and tolerated by either slowing the pace or by resting at intervals require only periodic observations. If the tissues of the feet are not involved or show only minimal changes, the patient is encouraged to exercise regularly. Special care in proper toenail cutting—allowing the nails to grow out beyond the flesh and then cutting straight across the nail—is followed. Avoidance of extremes of water temperature, immersing the feet in neither very hot nor cold water, prevents trauma to the sensitive tissues in this area and serious skin infections, which are likely to develop when the circulation is impaired.

Further damage to diseased blood vessels may result from the toxic effects of cigarettes. Cigarette smoking is especially dangerous in circulatory disease and must be stopped.

For persons who have symptoms of claudication that greatly limit normal activities, in whom symptoms are present even when they are sedentary, or in whom symptoms are progressively worsening, further diagnostic steps are indicated to determine the feasibility of operation. An injection of dye is made through a needle inserted in a peripheral artery, and x-rays are taken in rapid sequence to allow visualization of the involved peripheral vessels. Someone whose general medical condition is poor because of other serious illnesses should not be studied in this manner if surgical treatment is not planned.

If a blockage suitable for correction is found, a surgeon performs a bypass of the blocked area, using a synthetic graft to restore effective circulation around the blocked vessel. Another surgical procedure for peripheral vascular disease, which attempts to improve adequate circulation to the skin of the lower extremities, is a sympathectomy. This procedure consists of cutting the nerve trunks of the sympathetic nerve fibers. These fibers affect the tone and diameter of small arterioles, and their removal increases the diameter and hence the blood flow through them to tissues. Vasodilators, drugs that cause small blood vessels to dilate, may also be helpful in improving blood flow to the skin, but they are not generally effective in alleviating claudication.

Gangrene of an extremity requires a partial amputation to remove the dead tissue. The site of amputation depends on where healthy tissue starts, so that it may be performed at the mid-foot or above or below the knee.

Significant vascular disease can occur when other major blood vessels arising from the aorta produce circulatory impairment of the bowel and kidneys.

For reasons that are not completely clear, peripheral vascular disease seldom affects the blood vessels of the upper extremities to produce disease in the tissues or muscles of the arms. One exception is a disorder called Raynaud's disease.

Raynaud's disease refers to the constellation of signs and symptoms that some people, usually relatively young females, develop on exposure to cold temperature. During cold exposure, blood flow through our blood vessels is normally shunted away from vessels lying near the skin surface in order to decrease heat loss. The tone of our smaller blood vessels is controlled by nerve fibers from our sympathetic nerves, which vary the diameter of the blood vessels and, therefore, control blood flow. Persons with Raynaud's disease, on exposure to cold, have an exaggerated sympathetic nerve-mediated shunting of blood away from their fingers, toes, and nose leading to a blanching or whitening of the skin. This change may affect one, several, or all fingers. Upon exposure to a warmer temperature, the previously whitened fingers become purplish and red as the constricted blood vessels dilate, causing an increase in blood flow through them. Associated with the return of blood in these blood vessels is marked pain and discomfort. Some people with Raynaud's disease are quite incapacitated by the disorder. Some persons with this disorder even develop symptoms on removing something from a refrigerator. It may occur even in the summer, during gardening in cool soil. Although many people with this disorder have no other symptoms, it may develop in association with other diseases such as lupus erythematosus, rheumatoid arthritis, and scleroderma. In this setting it is called Raynaud's phenomenon. Patients who develop this disorder should seek medical help and be evaluated to exclude other disorders.

The treatment mainly involves efforts to avoid cold. Just as important is proper dress in cold weather to avoid triggering the signal to constrict blood vessels. At times, medications such as reserpine or guanethedine are given to block the nerve effect on blood vessels.

Aortic Aneurysm

The aorta must withstand the high pressure generated during each heartbeat. The constant thrust of blood under a mean pressure of 100 mm. of mercury contributes to the development of atherosclerosis on the interior lining of blood vessels. In addition, aging itself, as part of the general process of arteriosclerosis, causes the blood vessel to become more rigid and less elastic. Certain vulnerable persons develop a weakness in the muscle layer of the aorta. In a few cases, the weakness develops in association with other congenital defects in smooth muscle and connective tissue. The vessel wall undergoes progressive dilatation, causing either a cylindrical or a bubble-like ballooning called an aneurysm.

Aneurysms generally occur in older persons. An aortic aneurysm may cause relatively few symptoms and be detected during a routine examination by a physician who finds a prominent and widened pulsation in the abdomen. As the aneurysm enlarges, it causes pressure on adjacent organs and often leads to pain in the midback. The larger the aneurysm becomes, the greater the risk of rupture. A ruptured aneurysm causes bleeding and shock, and the patient usually dies.

The size of an aortic aneurysm can often be gauged on a plain x-ray of the abdomen. A useful technique for diagnosing the presence of an aneurysm is ultrasound. Ultrasound is a medical adaptation of a sonar technique developed during World War II to detect submarines. An instrument applied to the surface of the body directs high frequency sound to the body, bouncing off various internal structures and creating an image of different organs. The location, size, shape, and even density of organs can be accurately defined. Benign cysts can be distinguished from solid structures, which are more likely to be malignant. The procedure is painless and does not involve exposure to conventional x-rays. Once an aneurysm is suspected, dye is injected into the aorta to locate the defect accurately, to determine its exact size, and to note its relationship to other blood vessels, particularly the arteries to the kidneys. A surgeon trained in treating vascular disease can remove the aneurysm and insert a synthetic graft to restore the continuity of the vessel.

Most aneurysms of the aorta occur in the abdominal portion of the vessel. At times, the aneurysm can develop in the thoracic portion of the blood vessel. In this location, surgery is more complex because of the anatomical proximity to the heart and great vessels in the chest, which eventually supply the brain.

Diseases of Veins

Veins are the thin-walled blood vessels that return blood to the right atrium of the heart. There are two main venous trunks, the superior vena cava, which drains the upper extremities and the head, and the inferior vena cava, which brings blood from the legs and the abdomen.

Blood which leaves the heart in the aorta and other arteries, rich in oxygen, is returned by our veins with much of the oxygen extracted by the tissues of the body. In addition, most of our body acids generated during metabolism are carried in our venous blood and exhaled during breathing as a gas—carbon dioxide—in our lungs.

Unlike the blood pressure in the arterial system, which is high, the blood pressure in the venous circuit is quite low. Blood return to the heart from the upper torso is largely passive, and aided by gravity. Blood return from the lower extremities is all uphill, against gravity. The low pressure head in the venous system of the lower half of the body is aided by the presence of valves located within the veins; by negative pressure generated in the chest during inspiration, which draws blood upward; and by the leg muscles, which actually pump and squeeze blood through the veins during activity such as walking.

Almost all venous disease occurs in the venous channels located in our legs and pelvis. The two common disorders are varicose veins and phlebitis.

Varicose Veins

Of all the disorders of our circulation, varicose veins are the one of which most people are aware; we can see and feel them. Yet, they seldom cause significant problems.

There are two venous pathways carrying blood from the legs: the superficial veins, which travel on the surface of the leg, and deep veins, which lie deep within the tissues of the legs. Connecting or communicating veins link the deep venous channels to the superficial ones. If blood flow through our deep veins is impaired, blood is diverted by the communicating veins to the superficial ones. Disease in our deep veins, most commonly phlebitis or inflammation of the veins, increases the flow of blood through the superficial veins and increases the likelihood of varicose veins.

Veins are thin-walled and easily stretched. Varicose veins (tortuous, dilated veins) develop in many different situations. Certain persons inherit a tendency to varicose veins because of a weakness in the venous wall. Persons whose occupations involve much sitting or standing relatively immobile in one position, such as sales clerks, policemen, bus drivers, or dentists, tend to develop varicose veins. This is especially likely if previous disease of the deep veins has occurred so that venous return is already impaired. In addition to familial and occupational factors, pregnancy is a major cause of varicose veins. The increased abdominal pressure as the baby and uterus enlarge serves to impair venous return to a considerable degree and increase venous pressure, causing a dilation of the superficial veins. Women who have had several pregnancies generally have some degree of varicose veins, from a barely noticeable prominence to large, grape-like tortuous clumps of veins on the inner side of the lower leg and behind the knee.

Varicose veins usually cause little difficulty except for their appearance. When they become extremely large and tortuous, blood return is greatly impaired, blood forms stagnant pools, and, in time, leakage of blood cells forms areas of brownish pigmentation in the skin, especially around the ankles, called stasis dermatitis. The area tends to itch and be uncomfortable, and ulcers may develop, which heal quite slowly and tend to become infected.

Most people with mild varicose veins have no symptoms and need have little concern. Further progression of the disease can often be prevented by using elastic stockings or support hose to apply counter pressure and aid in the muscle pumping action and returning of blood to the heart. Efforts should be made to avoid sitting for prolonged periods of time. Elevating the legs on a footstool or hassock while sitting is encouraged as well as regular exercise, especially walking. Tight-fitting garments such as girdles or garters, which increase the venous pressure and retard blood flow, should not be worn.

For those who have large varicose veins or stasis ulcers that do not respond to local treatment, or who for cosmetic reasons wish them removed, venous ligation and stripping of the veins can be done by a surgeon. Generally, good results are achieved, but some persons with a susceptibility to varicose veins may develop new areas of varicose veins, especially if there is significant disease of the deep veins or if there are subsequent pregnancies.

Phlebitis and Blood Clots
Phlebitis, or thrombophlebitis, means inflammation of a vein. The commonest type of phlebitis occurs in the legs. Either the superficial or the deep veins may become inflamed.

Superficial phlebitis in the leg usually occurs because of an injury to the leg or irritation of the skin overlying a superficial vein, often in a varicose vein where the circulation is sluggish. The vessel and the nearby skin become tender to the touch, reddened, and inflamed.

Treatment of phlebitis involves elevation of the extremity,

application of hot moist packs to relieve inflammation, and, in some cases, use of specific anti-inflammatory drugs or antibiotics. The response is generally prompt, and no serious aftereffects develop.

Deep venous phlebitis is more insidious, since the vessels are not near the surface and the symptoms are often quite subtle. Most commonly, deep vein phlebitis occurs in hospitalized or bedridden patients who have been confined for a few days to several weeks. Often it develops in someone who is recovering uneventfully from an elective surgical procedure such as a hysterectomy or gallbladder operation. The combination of recent surgery and bedrest postoperatively is quite conducive to its development. Stasis, or sluggish blood flow, tends to occur in an immobilized or inactive person. Also, surgery tends to be accompanied by a hypercoagulable state, that is, blood is more likely to clot. Other predisposing factors include advanced age, obesity, tumors, congestive heart failure, and trauma to the legs.

For these reasons, patients who previously were confined to strict bedrest after surgery for weeks at a time are now often required to get up within one or two days in an attempt to prevent blood clots from forming in deep veins.

Deep vein phlebitis is most often first seen with pain. When a diagnosis of phlebitis is suspected, on the basis of certain physical findings in a patient who has had recent surgery, the physician sometimes attempts to document it by an x-ray of the venous channels, obtained by injecting dye or measuring the impedance of blood flow at the bedside. At times, phlebitis is discovered only when a blood clot has broken off from an inflamed vein and traveled to the heart and lungs— pulmonary embolus. A pulmonary embolus, if it is large enough, can cause sudden death or the picture of acute chest pain, cardiac failure, shortness of breath, or unexplained coughing up of blood.

Once deep vein phlebitis is suspected or documented, treatment is started with anticoagulant drugs to prevent further blood clot formation at the site of the inflamed vein while the body's defense mechanism digests already formed clots. Initially, the anticoagulant used is heparin, which is given intravenously at regular intervals. After a period of time, an oral type of anticoagulant is given—usually Coumadin, which takes the place of the intravenous heparin. Local measures, such as elevation of the legs and hot packs applied to the involved site, are also useful.

Prevention of deep vein phlebitis and its serious complication, blood clots, is most important. Early ambulation of post-surgical patients as well as the use of elastic stockings may be helpful. The use of heparin given subcutaneously in low doses can prevent blood clot formation in patients previously known to have had phlebitis, or in high risk patients such as those who have had orthopedic surgery, such as an operation for hip fracture. Even while lying in bed during the recovery from surgery and anesthesia, patients are encouraged to move their legs frequently.

Because of the increased risk for blood clot formation and pulmonary embolus, birth control pills should not be used by women who have had documented or suspected phlebitis.

Symptoms you should know about:

Chest pain.   Pain arising from the heart is usually in the middle of the chest, and it has a squeezing or pressing character. Angina pectoris comes on with exertion or emotion, and is usually relieved in a few minutes by rest. The pain of a heart attack may come on at any time and lasts longer. If you experience this, your doctor should be called, and if he is temporarily not available, you should go to your hospital's emergency room.

Shortness of breath.   When due to heart disease, shortness of breath occurs with exertion, but it may appear when you are lying flat so that it awakens you during the night.

Swollen ankles.   Swelling of ankles at the end of the day could mean congestive heart failure, although there are many other causes.

Palpitation.   This is simply the awareness of the heartbeat. Although sometimes frightening, it is usually not immediately serious and most often is not primarily due to heart disease.

High blood pressure.   As determined in public surveys or by the plant nurse, high blood pressure should always be investigated but is not an emergency.

THE LUNGS

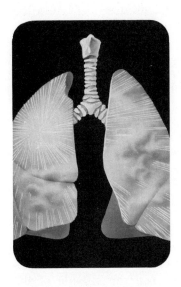

3

Normal Breathing (Respiration)
Breathing is a complex, coordinated effort involving the respiratory center in the brain, the muscles of the chest wall and diaphragm, the conduction of air through the airways, and finally the functioning of the lungs. The action is involuntary and occurs during sleep and activity. Even if we try, we can't hold our breath beyond a certain period of time. The frequency of breathing varies. A person may normally take eight to twelve breaths per minute and during exercise breathe two or three times as fast. The depth of breathing may vary from shallow breaths to a deep breath, as during a sigh. The volume of air inhaled and exhaled varies with the depth of breathing but usually averages 500 cc. (about a pint) of air in an adult.

The respiratory apparatus includes not only the lungs but also the nose, pharynx, larynx, trachea, and the structures of the chest wall—ribs and chest muscles and diaphragm. The function of the respiratory system is to provide enough oxygen to the tissues of the body both during a resting state, when needs are small, and during vigorous exercise, when the requirements increase several fold.

At sea level, the air we breathe contains approximately 20 percent oxygen, the rest being largely nitrogen, which is of no use to man, but necessary for plants. At higher altitudes, the oxygen content of air decreases, making it harder to breathe, especially for persons not used to such altitudes. Mexico City has a high altitude, and during the 1968 Olympics, many athletes from countries with lower altitudes performed less well than expected because of this problem.

The oxygen we breathe must traverse a series of branching airway tubes to reach the air sacs called alveoli with their network of tiny blood vessels called capillaries. Oxygen then is transferred through the alveolar wall by diffusion to red blood cells in the capillary bed. At the same time, carbon dioxide, a major waste product of body metabolism, is released from the red blood cells and diffused back into the alveoli and is blown out of the body during exhalation.

The lungs are in the chest on either side of the heart. (See illustration 4.) The right lung is divided into three main divisions, or lobes, and the left lung is usually composed of two lobes. A thin lining, called the pleura, covers the surfaces of the lung, and a space, the pleural space, separates the lung from the inner surfaces of the chest wall. The chest wall is composed of the ribs and muscle in front and back and the collar bone on top. An important muscle, the diaphragm, separates the chest and its contents from the abdominal cavity and forms the bottom of the chest cavity.

During inspiration, our chest wall muscles contract and lift the ribs outward; simultaneously, the diaphragm, sitting like a tent, is pulled downward, which pushes the abdominal contents away from the chest cavity. The outward lifting of the ribs and downward movement of the diaphragm create a pressure difference or gradient between the outside of the body and the chest cavity, which causes a movement of air into the lungs. The process reverses during exhalation. The ribs move back to their resting position, the diaphragm resumes its tent-shaped position, and air is forced out by the collapse of the chest wall and lungs as the degree of negative pressure generated during inspiration decreases. The movement of air in and out of the chest cavity is comparable to the action of a set of bellows.

Air is first drawn into the nose. The nose contains nerve endings concerned with smell. Anyone who, during a cold with a lot of nasal congestion, has experienced a loss of smell can appreciate the importance of this function. Even the desire for food, which is partially based on the fragrant aroma, can be affected by loss of smell.

The Lungs and Major Air Passages

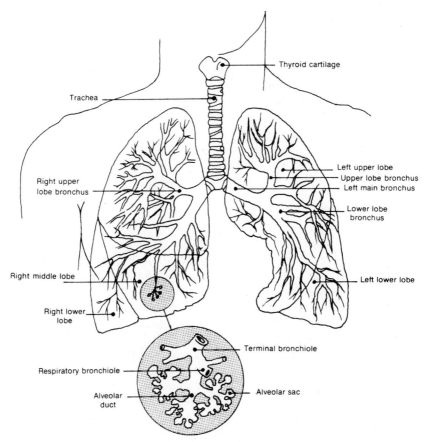

Illustration 4

The nose humidifies the air that passes through it, and this prevents excess drying and irritation to the tissues of the throat. People who snore often awake with sore, scratchy throats because of the drying effects of breathing air through the mouth, thus bypassing the humidification provided by the nose. Hairs in the nose serve to filter and purify the air by removing pollutants and particles.

Air then passes into the pharynx or back of the mouth, through the larynx or voice box, and into the trachea, located in the lower neck. The trachea, a large tube or airway composed of rings of cartilage, divides into two main airways, one for the right and one for the left lung. From the trachea about twenty divisions of the tubes occur, each dividing into two branches, which culminate in about 300 million air sacs or *alveoli* in the lungs. The initial tubes or airways are partially lined by cartilage, serving to maintain airway patency. These airways are called *bronchi*. Further down, at the eleventh division, cartilage is absent and the airways that conduct air toward the alveoli are known as *bronchioles*. Lining the airways are goblet cells, mucous glands, and cilia. The goblet cells and mucous glands form mucous secretions in response to irritation. The cilia or tiny hairlike structures act in concert, one after another, to propel foreign particles and mucus back toward the trachea and larynx, from where by coughing they are expelled as phlegm or sputum.

Respiration can be adversely affected by many different processes in any of the structures concerned with breathing. Adequate oxygenation of blood requires normal ventilation—involving the breathing center in the brain, spinal cord function, chest muscles, and diaphragm, patency of airways including nose, larynx, and bronchi, and the alveoli or lung tissue itself. In addition, normal perfusion of the lung by the blood requires a properly functioning heart and pulmonary blood vessels.

Diseases in the medulla of the brain, where the breathing center is located, may cause rapid death. Injury to the spinal cord or the nerve roots that control the muscles of respiration can seriously impair air movement or ventilation of the lung. A fracture of a vertebra in the neck can cause permanent injury to the spinal cord below the site of damage, causing paralysis of the limbs and inadequate ventilation because of loss of function of chest wall muscles and diaphragm. Poliomyelitis and amyotrophic lateral sclerosis (Lou Gehrig's disease) can affect breathing by injury to the nerve cells that innervate the muscles of respiration. Chronic allergy sufferers or those with a seasonal affliction may develop polyps in the nose, and these, together with boggy, inflamed nasal passages, prevent airflow through the nose. A piece of food or a small toy swallowed by a child may lodge in the larynx or voice box, obstructing the passage of air and causing asphyxiation and death unless quickly removed or dislodged. Acute disorders of the upper respiratory (nose, pharynx, or larynx) as well as lower respiratory tree (trachea, bronchi, or bronchioles) can interfere with breathing. These include viral and bacterial infections, inhalation of poisonous gases, and asthma. Chronic lung disorders, such as bronchitis and emphysema, may have acute flare-ups with a sudden deterioration of lung function. Breathing difficulties are a final expression of most heart diseases associated with congestive heart failure. Pulmonary emboli or blood clots may interfere with blood flow to the lungs, preventing adequate air exchange in the circulation, and producing a sensation of shortness of breath and labored breathing.

Shortness of Breath

A common problem patients discuss with their physicians is shortness of breath. Under average conditions breathing occurs with no specific awareness, proceeding quietly and imperceptibly.

Most of us are not in top physical shape, and we will experience a sensation of shortness of breath while climbing several flights of stairs or engaging in strenuous activities. Shortness of breath is the subjective feeling and awareness of labored or difficult breathing, accompanied by a heaving of the chest. An obese person may huff and puff even during regular activities because of the additional work of breathing imposed to satisfy his oxygen needs.

Shortness of breath cannot be measured quantitatively by the person experiencing it.

Persons with emotional and personal problems often complain of shortness of breath and a need to take deep breaths, almost as though their troubles add a weight to their chest and make breathing an extra effort. In addition, shortness of breath accompanies most lung ailments, including pneumonia, bronchitis, emphysema, and asthma, as well as severe anemia and heart disease.

Acute Bronchitis

Acute bronchitis is one of the commonest illnesses and usually is caused by a virus, such as the influenza virus, adenovirus, and Mycoplasma pneumonia virus. The suffix "itis" means inflammation. Bronchitis means inflammation of the bronchi (airway tubes).

The incidence of acute bronchitis parallels the increased incidence of respiratory infections during the winter months. Usually with the common cold, the upper respiratory passages, nose, throat, and larynx, are involved, but the lower respiratory system, including the bronchi, may also be involved. The lining of the bronchi becomes reddened, inflamed, and the mucus-secreting glands produce an excess of mucus. These changes result in coughing and expectorating mucous secretions, which may be yellow because of the presence of shed bronchial cells and white blood cells (pus).

Noxious gases, such as sulphur dioxide and chlorine, can irritate the bronchi and cause acute bronchitis. This problem can become serious in large urban areas, such as London and Los Angeles, where the concentration of harmful gases increases in association with smog or stagnant air that interferes with the normal cleansing of the air.

The average healthy person usually handles an episode of acute bronchitis without too much difficulty. The bronchitis may be part of an illness associated with other symptoms, such as headache, sore throat, nasal congestion, and muscle aches. Coughing is the hallmark of bronchitis. Initially, the cough may be dry and later be associated with mucus production or sputum. Slight discomfort of the chest and soreness around the breastbone may result from coughing. Persons with chronic lung diseases have an increased risk of developing complications from acute bronchitis. Their bronchi usually have anatomical abnormalities secondary to their chronic disease and are thus less able to handle the increased secretions caused by the acute episode. A superimposed bacterial infection producing pneumonia may occur and result in a further deterioration of the residual lung function.

Treatment for acute bronchitis is generally supportive. For the common viral illness, antibiotics are not beneficial. Fluids are useful to loosen secretions. Moist air provided by a humidifier is helpful as well as cough medications to loosen and thin bronchial secretions and aid in their expectoration. Codeine-containing cough syrups are useful to suppress nonproductive coughing—no sputum with resulting chest soreness due to the effort of coughing.

Chronic Bronchitis and Emphysema

Chronic bronchitis and emphysema, although two distinct disorders in their pure forms, commonly occur together so that the degree of disease caused by one or the other may be difficult to ascertain. Because the two disorders produce similar clinical pictures: shortness of breath, coughing, wheezing, and similar abnormalities of lung function, especially the obstruction to air flow during expiration, physicians refer to this family of diseases as *chronic obstructive lung disease.*

Emphysema is suspected by changes seen on a chest x-ray; large air cysts or bullae are noted as well as a low or flattened diaphragm. However, emphysema refers to the destruction of the walls or septae of the air spaces and the replacement of normal lung tissue by large air spaces. These pathological changes cannot accurately be determined during life and require postmortem study of the lungs. Emphysema is an anatomical diagnosis.

Pulmonary emphysema is seen more often in men over the age of 70 and in cigarette smokers. A high incidence of emphysema occurs in both sexes at a relatively young age in persons who have a deficiency of a serum protein, alpha-1-globulin antitrypsin.

Chronic bronchitis refers to excess mucus production, which results in the coughing up of mucus or sputum regularly. Increased numbers of mucus-secreting glands are present in the bronchi. The usual criteria for chronic bronchitis include sputum production daily for several consecutive months.

The most common cause of chronic bronchitis is cigarette smoking and the irritating effects of cigarette smoke. The smoker's cough, especially noticeable on awakening in the morning, is really chronic bronchitis.

Both chronic bronchitis and emphysema produce abnormalities of lung function of varying severity and reversibility. These disturbances of lung function can be determined by various breathing tests as well as by measurements of oxygen and carbon dioxide content in the blood.

The most consistent abnormality of lung function may be seen when a person tries to blow out all the air in his lungs after taking a deep breath. The increase in airway resistance

causes an increase in the work of breathing, leading to shortness of breath. The lungs are often overdistended, and
measurements show an increase in total lung volume. Another
feature is the unequal distribution of inspired air (gases), so
that some parts of the lung are poorly ventilated and others
receive adequate ventilation. Because the blood flow (perfusion) to these areas of lung remains undisturbed, the net result
is impaired oxygenation of blood, causing *hypoxemia*
(reduced oxygen content of arterial blood). Further lung
damage may lead to inadequate removal of carbon dioxide,
causing a retention of carbon dioxide in the blood, *hyper-
capnea*.

The severity of disease varies from person to person. One
patient may have minimal symptoms, with cough and sputum
production as the sole complaint and little progression of his
disease. Another may experience slowly increasing shortness
of breath over a period of several years. Far-advanced disease
may result in significant hypoxemia, so that even with
minimal activity or while at rest, shortness of breath is
marked.

As pointed out in the section on acute bronchitis, persons
with chronic lung disease are often in a precarious balance
regarding the ability to maintain adequate oxygenation of
blood. An acute disorder, such as a viral-triggered acute bronchitis, may significantly compromise their marginal lung
function and cause respiratory failure. A bacterial infection
commonly sets in because of the altered anatomical arrangement. The additional inflammation and damage to bronchi
causes further interference with air flow and distribution in
the lungs, so that the oxygen content of blood further decreases and a buildup of carbon dioxide levels may occur. As
the oxygen content falls and carbon dioxide is retained, the
patient's respiration becomes extremely labored and rapid in
the attempt to improve breathing and in response to air
hunger. The pulse becomes rapid, cyanosis or a blue
discoloration of the nailbeds and the lips develops due to
inadequate oxygenation of blood; lethargy, headache, and
even coma may ensue. The reduced oxygen content of blood
causes an increase in the pressure within the pulmonary circulation, which produces a strain on the heart and eventually
causes congestive heart failure. Chronic hypoxemia leads to
an increase in the number of red blood cells in the blood in
the body's attempt to increase the oxygen-carrying content of

blood. The resulting polycythemia, or thick blood, further increases the work of the heart and adds to the risk of heart failure.

Treatment of chronic obstructive lung disease is directed mainly at the reversible components, namely, the bronchitis. The anatomical changes produced by emphysema are permanent and irreversible.

The greatest effort is directed to avoiding irritants. For practical purposes, this means cigarette smoking. Every effort should be made to assist and encourage the smoker to stop smoking altogether. Other environmental pollutants should be avoided as much as possible.

Antibiotics are used to treat exacerbations of bronchitis, as the dangers of bacterial infections are great in these patients. Any change in the quantity or color of the sputum is an important sign and may indicate a serious change, such as a bacterial infection. The two common bacterial infections are due to Hemophilus influenza and the Pneumococcus organism.

Bronchodilators, such as ephedrine sulfate and aminophylline, can be useful in persons who have narrowed airways or bronchospasm as a component of their disease. Wheezing, which may be a prominent feature of chronic bronchitis, is also often relieved by these drugs that open up the airways. Mild sedatives are often given with these drugs to counter undesired stimulatory effects of the bronchodilators.

Adequate fluids are important to keep mucus secretions loose and easy to expectorate. Patients who do not respond to the above measures may progressively deteriorate, becoming increasingly hypoxemic, and may require hospitalization for intensive management. Therapy consists of intravenous fluids, antibiotics, the use of various types of mechanical respirators, and the frequent monitoring of arterial blood gases to gauge the effectiveness of treatment.

Bronchial Asthma, Hay Fever, and Allergy

Bronchial asthma is a common disorder affecting both sexes, all races and age groups, and often begins in childhood. The word asthma means a panting or shortness of breath, and anyone who has witnessed an asthmatic attack is familiar with the intense difficulty the patient has in breathing. Despite the availability of effective treatment, more than 4,000 deaths due to asthma occur annually in the United States.

Asthma is characterized by acute episodes of respiratory distress caused by certain precipitating factors, with disease-free intervals during which measurements of lung function can be completely normal.

Traditionally, asthma is divided into two types: those that can be related to an allergic response to an external substance—*extrinsic asthma,* and those that cannot be so linked but are probably a response to a respiratory infection, usually viral—*intrinsic asthma.*

Hay fever is quite similar to extrinsic or allergy-induced asthma and will also be discussed in this section. An understanding of allergy is relevant to both diseases.

Allergy. An allergy occurs when a substance, most commonly a foreign protein called an *antigen,* induces the body to form a protein directed against the antigen. This protein is called an antibody. Several different types of antibodies to challenge the antigen can be formed in the body by blood cells called lymphocytes. In an allergic response, the antigen reaches the target organ and is attacked by the antibody. In hay fever, the antigen is inhaled and affects the nasal passages, sinuses, and eyes; whereas in asthma the targets are the lower airways or bronchioles. The target organ literally becomes a battlefield as the body attempts to eradicate the antigen. The combination of the antigen and the antibody causes the release of several chemical mediators, including histamine, which set into motion the symptoms and signs of asthma or hay fever.

Frequently, the two conditions coexist in the patient, and most often there is a strong family history of both disorders. A person once subject to asthmatic attacks may see them completely disappear only to develop hay fever later.

The net effect of the allergic response in asthma is a swelling of the bronchioles and secretion of thick mucus plugs, which causes narrowing and obstruction of the airways. With hay fever, similar swelling and secretion of copious watery mucus occurs in the nasal passages.

Asthmatic attacks can be induced by various events, including temperature changes, emotional excitement, respiratory infections, strenuous physical activities, or exposure to a particular allergenic substance. Typical hay fever occurs in the early fall during the hay harvest when the pollen contaminates the air. However, other plants and grasses besides hay can cause similar "hay fever" symptoms at other times of the year when their pollens are present at appreciable levels. During the spring, trees, grasses, and flowers, such as roses, may cause inflammation of the eyes, nose, and sinuses as well as itching and a profuse watery secretion indistinguishable from classic hay fever. Later in the summer, ragweed causes a similar condition.

The common allergic substances or antigens are those that are inhaled and reach the lungs. Various pollens, grasses, mold spores, house dusts, industrial dusts (especially those from the processing of grains), flour, spices, organic solvents, such as glue, animal dander (or hair from cats, dogs, and horses), feathers, fabrics such as wool, and mattress stuffing, and many others are capable of inducing asthma in susceptible persons. Even a drug such as aspirin can cause asthma in a vulnerable patient.

During an asthmatic attack, air entry or inspiration is minimally affected at first; the narrowing of the airways caused by the mucus plugs and swelling makes expiration more difficult and prolonged, producing the wheezing sound, which, although the hallmark of asthma, does not exclusively occur in asthma. Wheezing is often audible to bystanders as well as to the patient. Because air entry is minimally affected but expiration impaired, overdistension of the lungs occurs. An asthmatic attack may be relatively mild and cause no derangement of lung function. But, as the degree of obstruction by mucus plugs becomes more advanced, the ability to provide adequate oxygenation of blood is impaired, causing a decrease in the oxygen content of the blood and air hunger. Finally, respiratory function may be so severely compromised that not only the degree of hypoxemia is great, but a build-up of carbon dioxide (the major waste acid product in the body) causes acid retention in the body leading to *respiratory acidosis*, a very serious condition, which can prove fatal if proper measures are not undertaken quickly.

The diagnosis of asthma can usually be made without difficulty by the physician. Generally, a family history of allergies is elicited, the patient has had previous attacks occurring at intervals with disease-free periods, and the physician can appreciate the characteristic wheezing and other chest findings. Laboratory studies can point to an asthmatic attack. A particular blood cell, the eosinophil, is present in higher numbers during allergic reactions. The sputum from the patient shows characteristic findings on microscopic examination.

Hay fever-like illnesses are easy to diagnose even for the layman. The person usually, but not always, has a seasonal affliction that is present at the time of year the particular pollen is prevalent in the air. The eyes are swollen, reddened, running, and itching. The nose is congested and full of mucous discharge due to congestion of the sinuses. Sneezing is often present, and the congestion and fluid formation causes discomfort behind the cheekbones and eyes. Headache is often present as well.

Skin testing is often useful during an asymptomatic period to establish the offending antigen both in hay fever and in extrinsic asthma. A battery of extracts of various substances is applied in very dilute concentration to the forearms either by injection into the skin or by scratching with a needle. The various antigens tested usually include pollens, grasses, trees, animal dander, molds, house dust, feathers, kapok, silk, wool, and various foods. An allergic response is evaluated by a physician or experienced nurse who gauges a positive reaction on the basis of the degree of swelling (wheal) and redness (flare). Properly performed allergy skin tests indicate the offending antigens and suggest the possible effectiveness of allergy injections. At times, positive skin tests, especially to food substances, are not reliable and represent a false positive reaction.

Treatment of asthma and hay fever can involve several different approaches. Prevention can be achieved in asthmatic persons if they avoid provoking substances; a person allergic to dog hair should not have a dog as a household pet. Allergy injections or attempts to desensitize may prevent the disturbance and can be very effective in hay fever sufferers whose symptoms are moderately severe and not controlled by the usual antihistamine drugs. Allergy injections can be beneficial in asthma patients who have extrinsic asthma.

At first glance, treating conditions caused by an allergic response to a substance by injections of the offending agent could seem contradictory. As indicated above, the symptoms of hay fever and extrinsic asthma result from the release of chemical mediators caused by the combination of antibody and antigen at the target organ. The antibody is produced by lymphocytes at the target organ that bind to various sites on the antigen. The rationale of allergy injection is to develop another antibody of a different class that combines and blocks the sites on the antigen. The allergic antibody no longer can combine with the antigen, since the binding sites are occupied by the blocking antibody. This is accomplished by giving allergy injections at regular intervals with increasing amounts of the antigen to build up a suitable level of blocking antibody. Allergy injections are beneficial to perhaps 50 percent of persons who receive them.

For asthmatic attacks that occur despite these allergy injections or in persons with intrinsic asthma, medicines are available. These drugs can reverse airway obstruction and improve airflow through the bronchioles. Two broad categories of drugs are used for asthmatic attacks: adrenergic agents and xanthine drugs. The former include epinephrine (adrenalin) and isoproterenol (Isuprel) and are available in tablets and in liquid form for use in nebulizers. Adrenalin is also given by subcutaneous injections. The xanthines include aminophylline and theophylline and are available in tablets, liquid forms, and rectal suppositories. For acute asthmatic attacks treated in the hospital, intravenous aminophyllin can be quite effective. Often an adrenerigic agent, a xanthine drug, and sedative are combined and are quite useful.

Recently, a new agent called cromolyn (Intal or Aarane) has been used to prevent asthmatic attacks; this drug is inhaled regularly and is effective.

Fluids to help loosen secretions as well as other chemical agents that thin secretions may be helpful. For asthmatic attacks refractory to these usual methods—adrenergic agents, xanthines, fluids, and antibiotics—steroids (cortisone-like drugs), which are anti-inflammatory agents, are used for several days. Some asthmatic persons may require long-term, low-dose treatment with steroids to prevent chronic and disabling asthma. A very effective steroid, which in proper doses avoids the systemic effects of oral steroids such as prednisone, has been developed in recent years for use as an inhalant in cases of asthma. Its name is beclomethasone and it is marketed as Vanceril. The use of this medication may enable control of severe asthma without any oral steroids, or with only small doses.

Persons with asthma who do not effectively respond to this treatment require hospitalization, vigorous therapy, and close monitoring of their response to treatment.

Often an asthmatic person who has visited an emergency room for several successive days is helped temporarily by treatment and discharged only to return several hours later in acute distress. The progressive fatigue, caused by the tremendous effort to breathe coupled with little sleep, makes hospitalization mandatory to initiate treatment to break the cycle.

Fortunately, most hay fever sufferers can be made comfortable by any of a number of antihistamine preparations whose main side effect is drowsiness.

Pneumonia

Pneumonia is an inflammation of the lung usually caused by an infectious organism, such as a bacteria or virus. Unusual causes of pneumonia, which together account for only a small percentage of cases, include chemical irritants, unusual drug reactions, and a host of other disorders.

Why pneumonia develops in an otherwise healthy person is a puzzle. Normally, the upper airway passages (nose and pharynx) contain numerous organisms that do not invade the lower airways and cause no harm. Pneumonia is likely to develop in certain persons who have predisposing causes such as chronic lung diseases (chronic bronchitis and emphysema) or whose lung tissue is abnormal, as discussed previously. Other vulnerable persons include postoperative patients, especially those who have had abdominal surgery and who are breathing abnormally in order to avoid pain and discomfort. Any debilitated patient who eats poorly or is unable to handle properly secretions that normally are swallowed (for example, a person with a severe stroke) may aspirate secretions from the stomach or mouth into the lung. Certain infants and young children who have defective antibody production due to an inherited disease of lymph node tissue as well as children with cystic fibrosis are very susceptible to pneumonia. Adults with acquired defective antibody formation, such as in chronic lymphocytic leukemia, are also prone to develop pneumonia. Pneumonia occurs frequently in terminally ill patients or in those with advanced cancer and in chronic alcoholics.

Many persons have been told by their physicians they have had pneumonia when in fact their illness was a bad cold or severe bronchitis. The term "walking pneumonia" has been used to describe either a mild pneumonia that requires no hospitalization or any other type of respiratory infection. Actually, a firm diagnosis of pneumonia should be based on chest x-ray confirmation of an infiltrate or abnormal lung shadow. A physician using a stethoscope can hear abnormal lung sounds over the appropriate chest wall area.

The pneumonia that is patchy and involves only a part of a lobe of the lung is called *bronchial pneumonia*. It may involve several parts of several lobes (often the picture in viral pneumonia). If an entire lobe is affected, it is called *lobar pneumonia*.

The clinical picture of pneumonia varies widely. The illness may begin as a cold-like illness but drag on with a persistent cough. On chest x-ray a patchy type of pneumonia can be identified. The patient may be first seen with chills, fever, purulent (pus) sputum, cough, shortness of breath, and chest pain. Sometimes the patient is quite ill and requires intensive care in the hospital to recover. Extensive viral pneumonia can interfere with oxygen transfer and cause life-threatening illness, as can a bacterial lobar pneumonia.

Approximately 20 to 25 percent of viral pneumonias will respond to broad spectrum antibiotics. The usual bacterial pneumonia in a nonhospitalized patient is caused by the pneumococcus and responds to penicillin. Culture of the sputum usually reveals the organism responsible for the infection and aids in selection of the appropriate antibiotic.

Before the antibiotic era, many persons died from pneumonia. The large number of antibiotics available today usually permits a cure of pneumonia in an otherwise uncomplicated case.

Pulmonary Embolism and Infarction
A pulmonary infarction follows a pulmonary embolus. An embolus is a blood clot that has broken off from the venous wall, traveled upstream via the main vein draining the lower part of the body, the inferior vena cava, to the right side of the heart, and then out into the lung through the pulmonary artery and its branches.

Blood clots usually form in the veins of the legs, but they may also form in the veins within the pelvis or abdomen, especially if surgery or recent pregnancy has occurred. The blood clot travels (embolizes) into the periphery of the pulmonary circulation, where the diameter of the blood vessels becomes progressively smaller, until it wedges in a pulmonary vessel—usually at a bifurcation or branching of the vessel. If the blockage is complete, the portion of lung served by that blood vessel undergoes injury, hemorrhage, and eventual tissue destruction or death, called an infarction.

A large pulmonary embolus can obstruct the pulmonary artery or one of its main branches, which causes acute obstruction of blood flow from the right ventricle of the heart; this may lead to a clinical picture of acute heart failure—shortness of breath, shock, and sudden death. A smaller blood clot travels farther into the periphery of the lung, traverses a series of smaller vessels until lodging, and blocks a blood vessel. If a pulmonary infarction occurs, blood and fibrin seep to the pleural surfaces, pleuritic chest pain and pleurisy develop, and hemoptysis—coughing up of blood—can occur.

The diagnosis of a classic pulmonary embolus with or without infarction usually is obvious to the physician. Characteristic chest x-ray and electrocardiographic changes can be present. However, a pulmonary embolus must be considered in any hospitalized or bedridden patient who has had recent surgery, a fracture, or a heart attack and who develops a rapid pulse rate, a drop in blood pressure, acute air hunger, shortness of breath, and heart failure.

Corroborative evidence of a pulmonary embolus can be obtained either by an abnormal lung scan or pulmonary angiogram. A lung scan involves injecting a radioactive substance into a vein and scanning the activity of the isotope on the surfaces of the lung. A clot in a pulmonary vessel causes decreased perfusion of blood flow in an area of the lung, and this supports a diagnosis of embolus. A pulmonary angiogram involves injecting a bolus of dye through a catheter threaded through a vein, usually in the arm, into the heart. A blocked pulmonary vessel shows as a cut-off of the dye due to the clot obstructing the vessel. An abnormal pulmonary angiogram is diagnostic of a pulmonary embolus. At times, the patient may be too ill and his condition too unstable for him to undergo transportation to the x-ray department or cardiology laboratory. Treatment for suspected pulmonary embolus should be initiated immediately—even while waiting for confirmatory laboratory tests.

Treatment of pulmonary embolus or infarction involves anticoagulation or blood thinning with the drug heparin, which is usually given intravenously. This drug prevents new clots from forming. Mechanisms exist within the body for digestion and removal of existing blood clots and pulmonary emboli. After control is achieved with heparin, oral anticoagulants can be given. Occasionally, despite adequate blood thinning with heparin, additional pulmonary emboli occur. In this circumstance, the inferior vena cava is tied off or ligated to prevent passage of blood clots from the legs and abdomen.

In several autopsy series, pulmonary emboli were found in a surprisingly high percentage of cases, most of which were not suspected during life. A suspicion of pulmonary embolus must be entertained at the proper time; delay of treatment often proves fatal.

Pleural Disease

Pleural diseases are relatively common, and the term pleurisy is used to encompass a variety of pleural disturbances. Pleuritic pain or discomfort is distinctive, since it is quite sharp and is aggravated by a deep breath or cough; the pain can literally "take your breath away," causing a person to take shallow breaths in order to avoid the pain. Not all pleuritic-type pain is due to pleural disease. Similar discomfort can also be caused by a strained chest wall muscle.

Many different disease processes produce pleuritic pain or pleurisy. Pleurisy is an inflammation of the pleura, which is a tissue that covers and lines the surfaces of the lung and inner chest wall. The relationship of the pleura, lung, and chest wall is best understood by imagining pushing your fist into an air-filled balloon. The fist represents part of a lung. The portion of the balloon in immediate contact with the fist is the *visceral pleura*, which has no nerve endings for pain. The outer part of the balloon represents the parietal pleura, which lies adjacent to the chest wall, and contains nerve endings for pain. The space between the visceral and parietal pleura, that is the air-filled space inside the balloon, is called the pleural space. Thus the source of pleuritic pain is the parietal pleura and not the visceral pleura.

Any disorder causing inflammation in the lung may involve the visceral and parietal pleura. Irritation to these surfaces causes fluid to form in the pleural space—a *pleural effusion*. If the inflammatory process involves the parietal pleura with its pain fibers, a deep breath allows the lung and visceral pleura to contact the surface of the parietal pleura, causing the sharp pain of pleurisy. If enough fluid forms to separate the two pleuras, pain may not be present. Pleural diseases may be secondary to other diseases, such as lung and heart ailments.

Pleural effusions commonly occur with heart failure. Pleurisy accompanies many lung infections, such as pneumonia and tuberculosis. Lung cancer often spreads to the pleura, causing pain or fluid formation. A pulmonary embolus, blood clot to the lung, can cause a pulmonary infarction, destruction of the lung and pleura, leading to pleuritic pain and effusion.

Primary pleural diseases occur less frequently than those listed above. The pleura can be involved in viral pneumonias in which the pleuritic pain predominates. A disease called epidemic pleurodynia is caused by a virus of the Coxsackie group and is associated with such severe pain that it is known as the "devil's grip." A pleural malignancy, called mesothelioma, occurs, usually with a history of previous exposure to asbestos. This disease is seen in asbestos miners, shipyard workers, and many others who have worked with materials containing asbestos, and may not appear for as many as 40 years after exposure.

Pleural diseases are suspected often by the description of pain related to the physician. Pleural effusions produce characteristic findings on examination of the lungs by a physician. X-rays confirm the presence of pleural fluid, and the fluid can be removed by insertion of a needle into the pleural space, a procedure called thoracentesis, or chest tap. Study of the fluid by various laboratory tests determines the cause of the fluid formation. Cultures of the fluid may confirm an infectious cause, such as a bacterial pneumonia, abscess, or tuberculosis. The fluid may show cancer cells or blood. The fluid formed in heart failure also has typical features.

Symptoms you should know about:

Cough. When cough is due to a mild upper respiratory infection, such as a cold or other virus disease, it usually does not last more than a week or so. Persistent cough should prompt a visit to the doctor.

Coughing up blood. When blood is coughed up, it can indicate a serious condition. It requires a doctor's examination, and usually, a chest x-ray.

Shortness of breath. Many things can cause shortness of breath, including lung disease, heart disease, and sometimes even anxiety.

Pain in the chest. Pleural pain ("pleurisy") arises in the covering of the lung, is sharp, and is aggravated by cough or a deep breath. A doctor should be seen for this condition.

THE GASTRO- INTESTINAL SYSTEM

4

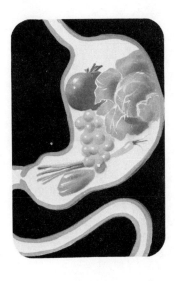

The Gas Syndrome

Everyone has experienced abdominal "gas" in one form or another—belching (doctors say "eructation"), bloating, gurgling, or passing gas by rectum ("flatus" in medical language). These complaints are among those physicians most commonly hear.

The gastrointestinal tract (or "gut," which is, believe it or not, a good word among even the most fastidious of doctors) is a distensible tube beginning with the stomach, continuing with the small bowel (or intestine) and ending with the large bowel and rectum. (See illustration 5.) The stomach begins the digestion of food. The starches, proteins, and fats we eat are broken down into simple sugars, amino acids, and absorbable fats; most of this process of digestion and absorption of these products into our body takes place in the small bowel. The large bowel participates in some further digestion and water absorption, and the liquid stool is formed into a solid residue in the final portions of the large bowel. Stool, or the formed bowel material, is largely composed of waste products, including fibers and residues of food particles that are not digested, bacterial products and bacteria, and shed or worn-out cells from the lining of the gut. Bacteria are normally present in our intestines and, in fact, are necessary for proper functioning of the bowel.

Diagram of the Gastrointestinal Tract

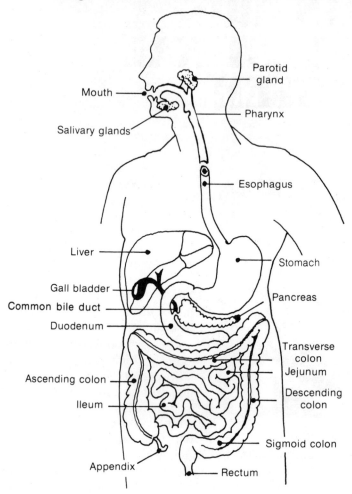

Illustration 5

We all remember from grade school days the mischievous child who could belch pretty much at will. He did this by swallowing enough air to distend his stomach and increase the pressure within the stomach to open the sphincter, or gate, which generally is a one-way door or passage into the stomach.

Most gas which is belched is due to swallowing air. We all swallow some air, especially when we eat and drink. Persons who are nervous and anxious tend to swallow greater amounts of air without realizing it. Cigarette smokers also tend to be air swallowers. Beverages that are carbonated produce bubbles of gas in our stomachs just as in a glass. Beer and soda drinkers have lots of gas in their stomachs and have a tendency to belch. Belching will occur as the balloon-like stomach distends and the pressure builds up, accompanied by a sensation of fullness and distress; this is relieved by the regurgitation of gas, which occurs during the belch. Bubbly, seltzer types of medications often relieve abdominal distress because they release bubbles of gas that distend the stomach and increase the pressure sufficiently to allow a belch and a relief of indigestion.

The stomach is connected to a long distensible tube, which twists and turns (the intestine) and ultimately ends in the rectum. Air can therefore pass through the stomach, into the small bowel, and eventually contribute to the formation of gas that is passed from the rectum. Gas that is finally expelled from the rectum can be a product of several different events. First, the passage of swallowed air or gas through the stomach and down the intestine, as discussed above, can cause flatus. Secondly, the fermentation of sugars by the bacteria in our bowel produces gas, just as yeast ferments grape juice into wine plus bubbles of gas. A group of researchers studied the mechanism of intestinal gas formation and found a correlation between the amount of gas produced by different persons and the number of bacteria residing in the bowel. Persons with large numbers of bacteria in the bowel produced greater amounts of gas than those whose bacterial counts were lower. We are all aware of certain foods—beans, cabbage, broccoli, and many others—that are notorious for producing gas as a by-product of their digestion.

Gas formed or swallowed has a tortuous journey through many loops of bowel. Often gas pockets are formed between columns of liquid or solid bowel contents, usually at turns and curves of the bowel tubes. These pockets distend the loop of the bowel and contribute to abdominal distress. Relief generally occurs with a passage of stool or expulsion of the gas from the bowel.

A certain amount of gas is a normal component of the digestive process. In fact, in certain cultures, such as the Arab-Bedouins, an appreciative guest signals to the host his pleasure for a fine meal by a hearty belch. In our society, we may try to reduce intestinal gas by avoiding gas-forming food and carbonated beverages. However, bacterial fermentation continues despite our wishes to the contrary. Our gut is outside of our body in a sense, so that in conditions of good health, the intestinal bacteria do not penetrate the rest of our body. These bacteria contribute to our health by aiding in digestion and forming useful products, such as vitamin K, which contributes to the production of essential clotting factors in our liver.

Belching, by opening the gate of the stomach, allows the acid stomach juices to reflux into the esophagus and cause heartburn—a chemical burn of the lower end of the esophagus. In this instance, antacids are effective for neutralizing the acid stomach contents. Despite much advertising and claims of effectiveness, there is no satisfactory medication in any form that significantly reduces gas formation or production. There are some measures that may disperse the gas or cut down on its volume. Certain medications act as detergents, spreading the gas throughout the intestinal tract, and decreasing the pressure areas that cause abdominal discomfort. Activated charcoal is taken as an adsorbing agent, that is, the charcoal actually adsorbs the gas and helps it pass through the intestinal tract without forming pockets. Persons with this problem should give up chewing gum and smoking and eat smaller amounts of foods that produce gas.

An important factor in reducing the discomfort of intestinal gas is the relief of tension. If the symptom is severe, tranquilizers may be used to decrease air swallowing. The intestinal tract will also be more relaxed with less pressure build up, and thus lessened discomfort from the gas that is present.

Constipation

It has been said that constipation is the heritage of civilization. Concern over the need for a daily bowel movement causes many visits to physicians' offices. Many body complaints as well as adverse emotional states are attributed to difficulty with bowel movements, not only irregularity but the size and shape of the movement. If we judge from the advertising media, much of our discussions with our friends involves our bowels. "You are only as young as you feel," implies that a laxative leading to a bowel movement will restore our vitality and zest for life.

From the earliest times of man, attention seems to have focused on bowels. The Ebers papyrus, written 3,500 years ago, recommends eating dates and using olive oil to relieve constipation. Efforts to rid the body of evil spirits, foul humors, and various diseases through vigorous purgings with laxatives have occupied a prominent role in the history of medicine—often contributing to or causing the death of a patient. The mystique of bowel movements and implied need for daily clockwork performance carries over into contemporary society. Many types of laxatives, pills, powders, liquids, health foods, fruits, and enema devices are used to stimulate bowel movements.

Just as we all look different externally, our internal machinery also functions differently. What one person may construe as diarrhea, another person might consider constipation. A story is told of a busy physician in the Maine backwoods who received a desperate call from a familiar patient, who had a long history of excessive complaints about his bowel movements. Interrupting before the patient could describe his symptoms, the doctor prescribed a strong laxative for "locked bowels." The patient objected and said he was having diarrhea and could not have locked bowels. The doctor replied, barely pausing in his answer, "Yes," he knew, "but it was locked in the open position."

The frequency of bowel movements is related to many factors, including amount of water, coffee, and tea consumed, and types of food and quantity consumed, as well as the inherent autonomic (involuntary) nervous control of the bowel. Some persons have one to three formed movements a day, whereas others function well with two or three bowel movements per week. The former patient does not have diarrhea, and the latter is not constipated, although the size and bulk of the bowel movements will be increased.

The chief complaint regarding bowel irregularity is constipation. The causes of constipation are multiple. One is a too hurried pace. Commonly, after a leisurely breakfast including warm beverages, milk, tea, or coffee, within 30 minutes or so a bowel reflex is stimulated, the urge to defecate is present, and a bowel movement can occur. But many of us eat no breakfast, or we dash to work or school and must suppress the urge to defecate.

Faulty habits are one of the main causes of constipation. A regular pattern of eating—three meals a day at relatively constant time intervals—tends to establish a regular pattern of defecation.

Constipation often occurs following a change in our routine, such as a trip out of town or a long plane ride. Many of us are somewhat fastidious and have become somewhat accustomed to the familiar surroundings of our own bathrooms or one at work. To use a bathroom on a train, in a bus terminal, or in a restaurant may not be satisfying, even though the urge to defecate is present, and a bowel movement is suppressed. Such suppression may cause constipation because the bulk or size of the movement increases and as water is lost through absorption in the large bowel, the stool hardens. Inadequate water intake also produces constipation, since the stools become hard.

Laxative users often become involved in a vicious cycle of diarrhea alternating with constipation. Concern over a day without defecation leads to the use of a laxative, which may empty the bowel by several loose, watery movements. Because of the cleansing of the bowel contents in this manner, it may take several days to form new residue and stool. The lack of a movement is interpreted as constipation and the cycle of laxatives repeated. Many patients follow such a routine for years.

Laxatives are of several main types, although hundreds line the shelves of our drugstores and supermarkets: irritants, bulk expanders, lubricants, and wetting agents.

The irritants work by their irritating effects on the bowel wall causing the intestinal contents to travel speedily through the small bowel, thereby preventing normal water absorption and presenting greater volume to the large bowel. They include castor oil, croton oil, cascara sagrada, senna, and phenolphthalein.

Bulk expanders are of two types. Some are salts that hasten the passage of liquid stool into the large bowel and retain large volumes of fluid which stimulate the urge to defecate. Epsom salts (magnesium sulfate), citrate of magnesia, and milk of magnesia are of this type. Constipation does result from our refined diets which contain little residue or bulk. Bulk expanders work by soaking up water in our bowel, and swelling in the process, and are not absorbed. Psyllium seed (Metamucil) and bran are of this type.

The lubricants or emollients, such as mineral oil, are non-digestible and nonabsorbable, and by lubricating the fecal contents, they prevent excess water loss and hardening in the large bowel.

Prunes, a household remedy for generations, combine many features of other laxatives, including bulk expansion, water retention, and direct bowel irritation.

Irritants in general should be avoided; in rare cases they can even contribute to perforation of the bowel. Lubricants are potentially harmful, especially in the elderly, where aspiration of the oil into the lung can occur and produce a type of pneumonia. Laxatives used excessively can cause electrolyte, or salt, disturbance in the body. Allergic reactions to laxatives have been described producing skin rashes, and a form of chronic hepatitis following the taking of certain types of laxatives has also been reported.

Many home remedies are used, often passed down from one generation to the next, and these are often effective, but, again are overused. Just allowing enough time for a leisurely breakfast with one or two cups of warm liquid, even water, often is very successful; this is nature's way! Fruits, such as prunes, which are laxatives, or bran-containing cereals which increase bulk, often help with bowel movements. Water intake, four to six glasses per day, keeps stools soft and makes evacuation simpler.

Sometimes, constipation occurs with disease processes in the rectum, such as hemorrhoids, fissures, or abscesses. The pain associated with passage of a bowel movement is sufficient to deter the urge to defecate, and constipation follows.

Inactivity is conducive to constipation, for it decreases the tone of the bowel. Bedrest may produce constipation, partially because of inactivity. Patients who are hospitalized and who are forced to use bedpans generally become constipated because of the general lack of enthusiasm and mechanical hardship involved in defecating in the supine position.

Physicians are very concerned about changes in bowel habits—not our established pattern of bowel movements. Recent changes in the size and shape of the formed stool or frequency of movement, or rectal bleeding in an adult over the age of 35 years, warrant thorough investigation by means of a digital rectal examination, proctosigmoidoscopy, and a barium enema. Cancer of the bowel is the most common cancer in the United States after skin cancer. A proctosigmoidoscopy allows the passage of a tube up to 10 inches into the rectum and visualization of the bowel wall. Up to 75 percent of all malignant growths can be seen with this instrument, and malignancies accompanied by changes of bowel habits are often located within this area. Sometimes they may be felt by the physician's finger. A barium enema allows for a complete visualization of the entire colon, especially above the range of the proctosigmoidoscope. By these means, the exact causes or source of the disturbance can be determined. Polyps or benign growths, hemorrhoids, fissures, inflammatory bowel disease, as well as malignant tumors can be diagnosed. If the tests are all normal, the patient can be adequately and convincingly reassured that all is well. In recent years, an instrument called the colonscope has permitted direct inspection of most of the colon; this is constructed of special optical fibers which transmit light, yet are so flexible they can be passed through the twists and turns of the colon.

Diarrhea

Diarrhea refers to multiple, loose, watery stools often accompanied by abdominal cramps. Diarrhea can be divided into acute and chronic disorders. Acute illnesses tend to be self-limiting and last from one to several days. Chronic disorders may occur for many months to years, and are often episodic with symptom-free intervals of varying lengths.

Acute Diarrhea. Attacks of acute diarrhea can result in dehydration and depletion of body salts. Young children are especially prone to have serious consequences from dehydration and require close supervision. The usual adult diarrhea accompanies an acute viral illness called gastroenteritis, usually lasting one to four days and which is self-limited. During the illness, treatment with bowel relaxants called anticholinergics is helpful. The diarrhea itself may be terminated by medications containing kaolin and pectate or opiates like paregoric. Fluids, tea and clear broth, should be given.

Diarrhea can be the main symptom of food poisoning. Food poisoning is usually caused by contamination with bacteria, the two common ones being Staphylococcus and Salmonella.

Staphylococcal food poisoning is usually due to contamination of dairy products and is especially common in warm weather, which allows bacterial proliferation. A typical episode might occur several hours after eating a cream puff or eclair or potato salad at the church bazaar. At times, many persons are infected, and the source of infection is determined by establishing what the victims ate in common. A rule of thumb is to eat creamed pastries and creamed foods only in months that contain the letter R in them (none in May through August) unless they are properly refrigerated.

Salmonella poisoning occurs commonly from eating poultry products, including eggs. A survey of poultry processing plants found a high percentage infected with Salmonella bacteria. Eating improperly cooked turkey, chicken, or raw eggs can cause this diarrheal disturbance, which occurs approximately 24 hours after ingestion of the contaminated food. Salmonella is quite common in small turtles purchased as household pets for young children, who may play with them and be exposed to the risk of infection.

Other bacterial infections can produce violent diarrheal illnesses accompanied by generalized effects, such as chills, fever, dehydration, and vascular collapse (a sudden drop in blood pressure to shock levels) with a significant mortality. These include cholera and typhoid fever. Fortunately, cholera is not found in the United States, and typhoid fever is quite uncommon. These diarrheal diseases occur as epidemics in underdeveloped countries and are usually spread because of stool contamination of the water supplies.

Diarrhea may also occur secondary to parasitic infestation of the gut. This condition is quite common in the tropics and underdeveloped areas as well as in the southern United States. This condition is established by finding the worm or, more commonly, its eggs in the stool.

A common form of diarrhea may follow the use of the broad spectrum antibiotics often given for treatment of an upper respiratory infection. The antibiotic kills many of the harmless bacteria that are normally in our gut, thus permitting the overgrowth of pathogenic or harmful bacteria which are not sensitive to the antibiotic and which produce diarrhea as a result of their overgrowth.

Certain antacids, such as Maalox, also are mild laxatives, and in large quantities can produce diarrhea.

Some persons develop allergy to milk and its products and are unable to metabolize the sugar in milk (lactose) and develop diarrhea on ingesting milk products. Many of these persons have learned to avoid milk products by trial and error. Drinking large amounts of coffee also may cause diarrhea. Stress can cause diarrhea in certain susceptible persons. This can occur, for example, before an important examination or an interview.

Travelers' diarrhea occurs in persons traveling to underdeveloped countries. In Mexico it is called tourista disease or, more appropriately, Montezuma's revenge. The cause is a toxin manufactured by certain strains of bacteria. It generally can be avoided by not drinking local water unless it is boiled, and by using only bottled beverages. Local produce, such as fresh fruit, should also be avoided.

The parasite Giardia lamblia is of worldwide distribution and is an occasional cause of traveler's diarrhea. Cases have been seen especially in persons recently returned from Russia. The diarrhea responds well to Flagyl or Atabrine tablets in 7 to 10 day courses.

Chronic Diarrhea.   Among the population of bowel sufferers is a distinct group of patients who are troubled with chronic lower bowel symptoms. They complain of recurrent diarrhea, which often alternates with periods of constipation. They experience vague abdominal pain under either the right or the left rib cage, often associated with gas and cramps. X-ray studies of the large bowel by a barium enema and the small intestine by a small bowel x-ray series, cultures of the stool for bacteria and ova and parasites, are all negative. This syndrome or symptom complex has been designated by many medical terms, such as colitis, spastic colon, functional bowel disease, or "irritable bowel syndrome," although no disease process can be identified. These patients tend to be very fastidious and somewhat rigid, overly concerned about bowel function, and have often tried all types of stool softeners, bulk expanders, and organic foods in an effort to resolve their difficulties. Many will reveal a cancer-phobia, and, despite reassurances, they go from doctor to doctor, including gastrointestinal specialists. Along the way, too many diagnostic x-ray procedures have been performed and together with various labels, such as spastic colitis, have reinforced a disease complex in the patient's mind. Some of these people have developed firm attitudes about the proper diet as well as the types of medication required to maintain a precarious bowel balance.

Another group of bowel disorders accompanied by diarrhea is the family of inflammatory bowel disease: *granulomatous colitis* or *regional enteritis* (Crohn's disease), and *ulcerative colitis*. Inflammatory bowel disease is an inflammatory process involving the inner lining or mucosa of the large bowel in ulcerative colitis, and, in Crohn's disease, involving all three coats of the bowel, mucosa, muscle, and serosa, of the small and large bowel.

These patients may be quite ill, depending on the degree of bowel involvement. Debilitating diarrhea, with as many as 15 to 20 movements a day, loose and watery with mucus and blood, may occur in association with violent cramps. The diarrhea may also occur during the night and awaken the patient. Weight loss and protein loss occur with various other complications, including anemia, joint disease, liver inflammation, as well as possible bowel perforation and fistula. Diagnosis is made after x-ray examination of the large and small bowel and proctosigmoidoscopy or colonoscopy, sometimes along with biopsy of the bowel.

Treatment varies with the extent of disease. Complete recovery may occur in ulcerative colitis with disease confined to the rectum. Nonabsorbable antibiotics, bowel sedatives and relaxants, and anti-inflammatory agents (steroids, etc.) are often effective. In certain cases, surgery with removal of the diseased part of the bowel is necessary to control the disease or its complications. These patients require the continued care of an internist or gastroenterologist for close follow-up and periodic examination of the bowel.

Another cause of chronic intermittent diarrhea or often an acute episode of diarrhea is *diverticulitis*. Diverticuli are small pouches ballooning off the bowel tube. The presence of these pouches is called diverticulosis and is a common finding in patients beyond the age of 50. Barium enema x-ray will reveal diverticulosis in almost all of the elderly. Diverticulitis occurs if one of these small pouches becomes infected or inflamed. Diarrhea may occur because of inflammation in the bowel. This condition is often accompanied by pain in the left lower part of the abdomen. Perforation of these inflamed pouches may occur, producing either a walled-off abscess in the abdomen or a generalized infection called peritonitis. Treatment is usually effective with antibiotics; in some cases, intravenous fluids must be given and the bowel rested by not allowing the patient to take food or liquid by mouth until the process subsides. Surgical intervention sometimes becomes necessary to remove the diseased or involved portion of the bowel or to divert fecal material away from this area. A low roughage diet, one with minimal food residues or fibers—no fresh fruits or vegetables—often is helpful in patients who have inflammatory bowel disease. However, such a diet is used only in the acute inflammatory stage, and it is currently felt that a diet low in fiber is the cause of diverticulosis. This is the reason diverticulosis is so common in civilized nations where the diet is based on refined starches and contains less fiber for stool bulk.

Peptic Ulcers

What is an ulcer? The word ulcer means simply a localized erosion of a surface. Such a process is fairly common in the gastrointestinal tract, where the lining is eroded, or ulcerated, exposing the underlying fibrous and muscular tissue. This ulceration is usually associated with some inflammation of its base and the surrounding tissues, and with spasm, or tightness of the muscles, in that portion of the stomach or intestine. Although an ulcer can occur in any portion of the intestine, almost all ulcers that produce symptoms are located either in the first part of the small intestine called the duodenum (duodenal ulcer), or in the stomach itself (gastric ulcer).

Normally, the stomach secretes hydrochloric acid and gastric juices containing enzymes such as pepsin, which start the digestion of foods. Because excessive acid and pepsin secretion are associated with duodenal ulcers, they are called peptic ulcers. Why the stomach itself is not digested by its own secretions remains a mystery. It may be that a mucous coat or film lining the surface of the stomach serves as a sufficient barrier under normal conditions, and an ulcer may represent a breakdown of the protection by factors yet to be identified.

Ulcers are common and most occur in the duodenum. It is estimated that approximately 10 percent of males develop a duodenal ulcer during their lifetime. Persons with duodenal ulcers generally produce excess amounts of hydrochloric acid, whereas gastric ulcers are often not related to excess acid production.

Patients most often seek medical attention for relief of abdominal distress or pain. The diagnosis of a peptic ulcer may be straightforward; but sometimes other disorders, such as gallblader disease, hiatal hernia, esophagitis, or air swallowing with bloating, belching, and heartburn may be possible diagnoses from the description offered by the patient.

Usually, a gnawing pain, localized to a small area in the epigastrium (midway between the end of the breastbone and belly button) is described. The pain generally occurs several hours after eating when acid production is increased and can even awaken the person from his sleep. Milk, food, and antacids often provide temporary relief. Depending on the location of the ulcer, the pain may radiate straight through to the back.

What causes an ulcer? Certain factors predispose to ulcer formation. Ulcers are more apt to occur in hard driving, ambitious persons who are under stress and pressure. Some ulcer patients appear unable to release their anger and frustration in usual ways, such as a burst of yelling or ill temper; they readily admit to "holding it in" and are unable to "let it out."

Our brain, via a large nerve called the vagus nerve, is able to stimulate and augment acid production in the stomach. The Russian physiologist, Pavlov, demonstrated conclusively the role of conditioning and expectation on gastric acid production. Dogs were fed in association with stimuli, such as bells and lights. After a period of time, they were shown to produce an increase in gastric acid with the appropriate stimulus even though food was withheld. Even the smell of food causes increased acid production in the stomach. The central nervous system, subject to the influence of our feelings and emotions, mediated by the vagus nerve, thus can influence gastric acid production. As William James said, "The Lord may forgive our sins, but the nervous system never does."

Alcohol is a potent stimulus to acid production, and since duodenal ulcers do occur in situations of excess acid production, alcohol may be a provoking factor. In addition, alcoholic beverages directly irritate the stomach lining.

Certain types of food, especially spicy and highly seasoned foods, are associated with increased acid production. Caffeine-containing beverages, such as coffee and tea, and cola-containing carbonated beverages are associated with increased levels of stomach acid. However, even decaffeinated coffee causes an increase in stomach acid production, which indicates that other unidentified constituents of coffee besides caffeine play a role.

Many drugs that are prescribed for various illnesses may also be ulcerogenic. Aspirin-containing drugs may also be associated with ulcers and should be used cautiously by persons with previous ulcer disease, and avoided by patients with active ulcer disease. Persons using large amounts of aspirin for chronic illnesses, such as rheumatoid arthritis, are candidates for gastric or duodenal ulcers. Buffering of aspirin does not prevent this danger. Other commonly used drugs associated with ulcer include reserpine-type drugs, used for control of hypertension, phenylbutazone (Butazolidine), used to treat bursitis and inflamed joints, and steroid preparations, such as cortisone, used in a number of disease states.

Ulcers occur in greater numbers in persons who have some unusual types of tumors. Persons with a tumor of the parathyroid gland, which regulates the level of the calcium in the blood, have a higher incidence of peptic ulcers. A rare cause of ulcer disease is a tumor of the pancreas associated with the production of a hormone called gastrin, which is a potent stimulus of acid production in the stomach.

Complications.   Ulcers may cause other problems besides abdominal pain. They may erode into a blood vessel and produce bleeding, so-called bleeding ulcers. If the blood vessel is a large one, the bleeding may be brisk, and the person may vomit blood and pass bloody or tarlike stools. If the bleeding is gradual or intermittent, symptoms of anemia with weakness and tiredness may be the main problem. The person with a bleeding ulcer may be aware of a darkening of his stools, which may be black in color.

If the ulcer is large, and penetrates through the entire wall of the stomach or duodenum, a perforated ulcer is present. The stomach juices and acid spill into the abdominal cavity, the digestive enzymes produce a chemical irritation called *peritonitis*, associated with severe pain, a board-like or rigid abdomen, and shock. Such a patient requires immediate hospitalization and surgical intervention.

Persons who have had repeated episodes of ulcers may develop narrowing between the stomach and duodenum by scar tissue, producing obstruction to the emptying of the stomach. Vomiting of undigested food occurs, and in time significant weight loss. Surgery is required to correct blockage or obstruction so that normal digestion may occur.

Diagnosis.   Once a patient discusses his problem with his doctor, x-rays of the upper gastrointestinal tract—an "upper G.I. series"—are often obtained to establish the diagnosis and locate the site of the ulcer.

This sort of study is carried out by a radiologist, a doctor who specializes in x-ray interpretation and treatment. Since the stomach and duodenum have the same x-ray density as the other organs and tissues in the abdomen, they ordinarily don't stand out when a plain x-ray picture is taken. However, if the subject swallows a radio-opaque substance, such as barium sulfate, this is easily seen on x-ray study, and since it conforms to the shape of its containing vessel—in this case, the stomach and duodenum—it gives a good picture of the upper gastrointestinal tract. Such an examination must, of course, be carried out when the patient has an empty stomach.

Duodenal ulcers are always benign. If the symptoms improve and disappear on treatment, no further studies are necessary. Gastric ulcers may be malignant, or cancerous, in a small number of cases. Therefore, after a period of treatment, even if the symptoms improve or disappear, repeat x-rays of the stomach are obtained to see healing and complete disappearance of the gastric ulcer. Gastric ulcers are also studied by means of a fiberoptic instrument called a gastroscope, which is a flexible tube swallowed by the patient and passed into the stomach. The gastroenterologist who does this procedure can see the gastric ulcer and get a good idea whether it is benign or malignant. To confirm his impression, he often will biopsy, or snip off, several surfaces of the ulcer wall and submit the tissue and washing from the ulcer to a pathologist, who will examine them under a microscope.

Treatment.   The treatment of ulcer disease is usually by medical methods and not by surgery. Hospitalization of ulcer patients is generally unnecessary except in cases of bleeding or perforation. Persons with bleeding ulcers require close monitoring and transfusions to support the circulation and avoid shock. Surgery becomes necessary when the bleeding continues despite efforts to control it or if the bleeding is excessive. As stated above, perforation of an ulcer requires prompt surgical intervention.

Symptoms of obstruction are usually gradual and if associated with an active ulcer, may respond to medical, nonsurgical, management. If the ulcer is chronic and refractory to treatment, surgery is indicated.

Occasionally, an ulcer fails to heal while the patient is on medical therapy at home; for this reason, he may be hospitalized for optimal sedation and environmental control— limiting visitors and controlling activity levels. However, for most ulcer patients, staying at home is adequate for healing of an ulcer on a medical program.

The usual diet for an active peptic ulcer is bland, which means avoiding spicy and fried foods, and relying heavily on dairy products, broiled meats, cereals, and creamed-type foods. Since duodenal ulcers are associated with acid production, efforts to neutralize acid are the mainstay of therapy. Food is a good neutralizer of acid and, therefore, frequent feedings are recommended. Antacids, chemicals such as aluminum hydroxide and calcium carbonate, are taken frequently to neutralize gastric acid. These and other antacids are present in many commercial preparations, such as Maalox, Gelusil, Mylanta, Di-Gel, Camalox, etc.

By and large, these have similar antacid properties, and differ only by the addition of mild cathartics or agents to disperse gas. These antacids are nonabsorbable, that is, they can be used in large amounts because they do not pass into the blood stream, but rather just move through the intestine after they have neutralized the stomach acids. Absorbable antacids, however, such as baking soda, Sippy powders, and Alka-Seltzer, can alkalinize the system and cause serious side effects if taken in too large quantities.

Medications, called anticholinergics, are given to inhibit acid release from the stomach. Tincture of belladonna is a well-known chemical used to inhibit acid secretion. Belladonna, or a derivative, or a similarly acting drug is present in many different medications prescribed for the treatment of peptic ulcer disease, such as Donnatol, Belladenal, Probanthine, Dartal, and many others. Besides inhibiting acid production, these medications also relax an abnormally tight stomach or intestine. They are used for other conditions besides peptic ulcer disease, where gastrointestinal spasm is present. They have still other effects, which makes them dangerous to use in persons who have glaucoma or urinary retention. The drug cimetidine (trade name Tagamet) effectively stops the secretion of acid in the resting stomach, and cuts down acid production in response to stimulation by food to less than one-third of the normal amount. This, of course, makes it valuable in the treatment of peptic ulcer patients.

Side effects of cimetidine are not common, but for long-term use antacids are safer and probably as effective. Cimetidine is most valuable in the initial treatment of new cases of duodenal ulcer.

Alcoholic beverages, coffee and tea, and certain classes of drugs cited above are avoided. Patients are encouraged to minimize external conflicts and worries as best as possible. Mild sedatives or tranquilizers are extremely useful in reducing anxiety and establishing a restful milieu.

Once an ulcer has healed—and ulcers may heal rapidly, even in just a few days—the person may gradually return to his former activity level and resume a normal diet. If precipitating factors were present (certain medicines or excessive consumption of alcohol), these must be avoided to prevent a recurrence. Diet should be individualized, and one's own experience guide the selection of foods. The person with a history of ulcers should avoid foods that consistently upset his stomach or cause indigestion or heartburn. Many people can resume a diet with spicy and well-seasoned foods with little difficulty.

For patients who require surgery, different operative procedures are performed depending on the particular complication—bleeding, perforation, or obstruction. To some extent, the surgical method also reflects the personal bias of the individual surgeon, depending on his own training and experience. The surgeon achieves the greatest success with the procedure with which he is most familiar.

Surgeons generally are moving away from gastric resection—the removal of 50 to 75 percent of the stomach. The procedure makes good sense, for it removes the antrum of the stomach that produces gastrin, which stimulates acid production, as well as the fundus and body of the stomach where acid is secreted. However, with the removal of a large portion of the stomach many persons can eat only small amounts before becoming full and uncomfortable. A large weight loss may occur. After eating, the food is rapidly dumped into the intestine, producing diarrhea as well as symptoms of weakness, sweating, and headache, especially following a meal with carbohydrates—the so-called dumping syndrome. Many surgeons now perform a *pyloroplasty*, widening the opening of the channel from the stomach, so food cannot stay as long in the stomach and stimulate acid release, combined with *vagotomy*, cutting the vagus nerve.

Gallbladder Disease

Medical students are taught to consider gallbladder disease in the differential diagnosis of indigestion, dietary distress, or abdominal pain, especially if the person is "female, fair, fat, and forty." Gallbladder disease is common and affects both sexes, increases in incidence with advancing age, and is not limited to blonds. Gallstones occur in approximately 20 percent of persons over the age of forty.

The Normal Gallbladder. The gallbladder is a bag or reservoir about the size of a pear, which lies under the liver and which stores and concentrates bile. Bile is formed in the liver and transported by bile ducts into the gallbladder. It is a golden brown fluid composed of bile salts, bile acids, pigments such as bilirubin, and cholesterol.

During the process of digestion, the acid stomach contents reach the small bowel—duodenum and jejunum—and cause the release of an enzyme called cholecystokinin. Cholecystokinin stimulates the gallbladder to contract and discharge its contents of bile into a channel called the common bile duct, bringing the bile into the duodenum and small bowel. The bile salts and acids aid in the absorption and digestion of dietary fats as well as vitamins A, D, and K, which are not water soluble.

What are Gallstones? Gallstones are concretions composed of pure cholesterol, inorganic calcium salts, bilirubin, cellular debris, or any combination of these. Stasis, or stagnation, of bile in the gallbladder predisposes to the forming of small crystals and eventual stone formation. This may be the mechanism for stone formation in pregnancy and in prolonged fasting or starvation. Cholesterol remains dissolved in solution largely by the action of bile acids and if the concentration or ratio of bile acids decreases, cholesterol crystals may precipitate and eventually form a stone. Cholesterol stones tend to be yellow-white in color, whereas bilirubin stones are black. Gallstones may be multiple or single; they may be as small as salt granules or as large as a hen's egg.

Symptoms. Persons with gallstones may be perfectly asymptomatic or have a variety of symptoms and complaints that cause them to seek medical assistance. Nausea, flatulence, belching and indigestion may be prominent. Because of these symptoms a physician may suspect gallbladder disease and order x-rays of the gallbladder as well as an upper gastrointestinal series to rule out other disorders such as ulcer disease or a hiatal hernia. Gallbladder x-rays are obtained by having the patient ingest iodine-containing tablets the evening before the x-ray. These tablets are absorbed from the intestine into the liver, where they are excreted into the bile, and concentrated by the gallbladder. If the gallbladder is diseased, no dye is concentrated and the gallbladder may not visualize. If gallstones are present, they appear as shadows contrasted with the opaque dye. Ultrasound, mentioned in the section on aortic aneurysm, is very accurate in detecting gallbladder disease.

Even if gallstones are present, it is not always certain that all the symptoms complained of are due to them and after removal of the diseased gallbladder, various symptoms really unrelated to the gallbladder may persist.

Discomfort after meals, usually located under the lower right ribs extending around to the back, may be present. This distress may occur with rich foods that contain a lot of fat, such as fried and greasy foods, gravies, and dairy products, such as milk, ice cream, and cream. Fatty foods stimulate the gallbladder to contract, and if stones are present, they may wedge into the outlet of the gallbladder and produce an acute gallbladder attack, characterized by nausea, vomiting, and severe cramping pain. If a stone is pushed into the bile common duct and becomes impacted, obstructing the flow of bile, acute inflammation of the common duct occurs, which may produce high fever, chills, and vomiting; the attack may be associated with jaundice and yellowing of the eyes secondary to obstruction of the flow of bile from the liver.

Gallbladder attacks may range all the way from the feeling of indigestion or abdominal distress after meals that occurs with dietary indiscretion to episodes that bring an acutely ill person to the hospital and emergency surgery to remove the swollen inflamed gallbladder and stone or stones blocking the common duct.

Treatment.   When disease of the gallbladder is diagnosed, even if the person is relatively asymptomatic, gallbladder surgery is generally recommended. The gallbladder is not necessary for good health or proper digestion. Gallbladder removal is elective surgery and can be done at a convenient time, with any factors that may possibly increase the risk of surgery properly evaluated and corrected. Gallstones do not disappear. Even though recent attempts to dissolve them by chemicals appear promising, such efforts currently remain experimental.

Gallstones predispose to the small additional risk of cancer of the gallbladder.

Gallstones may, by lodging in the common duct and by obstructing the bile passage, produce serious liver damage. The political career of Sir Anthony Eden, former Prime Minister of Great Britain, was terminated by illness resulting from gallbladder disease and inflammation of the common duct.

Pancreas

The pancreas is an important organ, located deep in the abdomen behind the stomach and wedged in the concavity formed by the sweep of the duodenum (the first part of the small bowel) and extending over to the spleen. (See illustration 5.) This gland produces the important hormone insulin, so vital for fat and sugar metabolism (see the section on diabetes mellitus). Other hormones, such as glucagon, are also made in the pancreas.

The pancreas also provides important digestive enzymes necessary for the absorption of carbohydrates, protein, and fat from our diet. Pancreatic secretions are stimulated by intestinal enzymes released upon contact of the partially digested food passing from the stomach into the small intestine. The pancreatic secretions are alkaline, and they neutralize the acid stomach contents passing into the small bowel, which could otherwise injure the lining of the intestine.

Pancreatic enzymes participate in the process of digestion by converting food into forms that can be assimilated and absorbed by the small intestine. Carbohydrates are broken down into simple sugars, protein is split into fragments called peptides, and together with bile salts produced by the liver, pancreatic enzymes convert fat to fatty acids.

Acute inflammation of the pancreas, *pancreatitis*, has various causes and the patient is usually first seen with abdominal pain, nausea, vomiting, and even shock. Patients with acute pancreatitis are often extremely ill. The picture may resemble an acute gallbladder attack, a perforated ulcer, or even a heart attack.

Acute pancreatitis is often seen with gallbladder disease. A stone from the gallbladder can lodge in the common bile duct, and since in 70 percent of people the pancreatic duct joins the common duct before entering the duodenum, a stone can block the duct and cause a build-up of back pressure in the pancreas, thus producing acute pancreatic inflammation.

Another commonly associated cause of acute pancreatitis is excess use of alcohol. Pancreatitis may also be caused by viruses, such as mumps. Very often no clear cause can be identified.

The diagnosis is usually established by finding an elevation of certain pancreatic enzymes in the blood or urine called amylase or lipase. The other diseases that have the same symptoms as pancreatitis have to be excluded. Surgical intervention for an acute gallbladder attack is quite beneficial, but if the patient really has acute pancreatitis, it may be disastrous.

Most cases of pancreatitis resolve with such measures as pain medication, emptying the stomach by suction through a tube, and maintaining fluid needs by intravenous feeding while the patient remains fasting. Repeated attacks of pancreatitis gradually cause scarring and calcification in the organ, resulting in abnormal pancreatic function.

Chronic pancreatitis. Diseases of the pancreas can interfere with the process of digestion and produce poor absorption, especially of fat. Weight loss, vitamin deficiencies, and the passage of voluminous stools with large amounts of fat, or steatorrhea, can result from inflammation and injury to the pancreas. Diabetes mellitus also develops when sufficient pancreatic tissue has been damaged.

The digestive disturbances can be improved by using tablets that contain pancreatic enzymes, and injections of insulin control the symptoms of diabetes mellitus.

Cancer of the pancreas appears to be increasing in frequency. Most often it escapes recognition until the disease is advanced and chances of cure by surgery are quite small, and currently chemotherapy only helps a fraction of the patients.

Liver Disease

The human liver is certainly an unappealing organ. It is a large, purplish-brown mass high in the right side of the abdomen; cut sections look like the calf's liver for sale in the butcher shop. Yet this homogeneous tissue is a fascinating chemical factory that performs many functions essential to life. The removal of the liver causes death just as surely as removal of the heart, brain, or both kidneys.

The liver forms and secretes bile, which helps digestion and rids the body of worn-out cell pigment. Many proteins are manufactured in the liver, including the albumin in our blood and many of the factors important in blood clotting. Thousands of different enzymes are necessary for all the chemical reactions that take place in the liver, and these have to be made on the spot by the liver cells. Breakdown of amino acids takes place in the liver, urea synthesis, and the making of fats, including cholesterol. Glucose is stored in the liver, and its availability is important in regulating the blood sugar. Through several different mechanisms, the liver is able to protect us against poisonous substances made in the body or taken in as food and drink. Many of the drugs we use are chemically altered in the liver.

More than enough cells are present in the liver to carry out these various jobs, so that even if a large volume of liver is lost, the function can still be satisfactory. Many diseases can involve the liver, and the organ reacts largely by two forms of damage—hepatitis and cirrhosis. *Hepatitis* means inflammation of the liver and is a reaction to cell injury or cell death caused by a virus or drug. Viral hepatitis is discussed at length elsewhere in this book. *Cirrhosis* is a more chronic process, that is, one that takes longer to develop, and is characterized by death and loss of liver cells, thick scars, and small clumps of newly growing liver cells. These changes make the cirrhotic liver lighter in color and irregular, with a nodular surface.

There are several types of cirrhosis. Biliary cirrhosis results from longstanding blockage of the bile ducts, either within the liver or after the large collecting tubes leave the organ. Hemochromatosis is a form of cirrhosis that is caused by excessive iron deposits in the liver. Cardiac cirrhosis occurs in patients with heart failure after chronic congestion of the blood vessels in the organ has caused damage to the liver. Other rare types are due to several sorts of congenital flaws. An increasingly common type of cirrhosis in America, and probably the most frequent type throughout the world, is postnecrotic cirrhosis; it may follow viral hepatitis, poisoning with industrial chemicals or drugs, or certain infections that are unusual in our country. The most common type of cirrhosis in America and most of western Europe now is portal cirrhosis.

Portal Cirrhosis.   Chronic alcoholism is the major cause of portal cirrhosis. About 75 percent of patients with this disease admit to heavy drinking, and it is estimated that between 10 and 20 percent of all known chronic alcoholics have cirrhosis.

It used to be thought that dietary deficiencies of certain vitamins and proteins was the cause and that alcoholics were
susceptible because of their poor nutrition. We know now,
however, that alcohol itself can cause liver damage that
leads to cirrhosis. Even a well-nourished alcoholic can develop portal cirrhosis. It seems reasonable that malnutrition
contributes to the development of this condition in those alcoholics who eat poorly. In the cases of portal cirrhosis that
are not associated with long-term alcohol abuse, doctors do
not know the cause.

Cirrhosis occurs a little more frequently in men than in
women and usually becomes apparent in middle age. A few
persons may have cirrhosis and not be aware of it. The doctor
occasionally finds this disease on routine examinations in
persons who consider themselves well. This is unusual,
however, and when evidence of liver disease is picked up in
this manner, it is usually a completely curable precursor state,
called fatty infiltration of the liver. Although the liver is
enlarged in these persons and liver function tests are abnormal, they have not yet passed into the stage of cirrhosis.
Stopping the use of alcoholic beverages and establishing
normal nutrition result in complete reversal of the process.
Over a period of many months, the liver returns to a normal
size and the blood tests become normal.

Most persons who have portal cirrhosis feel sick. The
disease begins insidiously, with weakness, loss of appetite,
vague indigestion, and easy fatigability. In several months'
time the victim may begin to lose weight and then notice
enlargement of his abdomen and an off-and-on swelling of his
ankles in the evening, which disappears after a night's sleep.
He feels sick, and his family and friends begin to think he
looks ill.

He may suddenly worsen after an especially big drinking
bout, or he may slowly go down-hill in a period of several
years. The development of jaundice, large amounts of fluid in
the abdomen, or mental changes signify serious liver failure.

Jaundice comes about in patients with cirrhosis when the
liver is unable to excrete the blood pigments, and they accumulate in the blood and then in the various body tissues,
where they cause a yellow color. This is usually first noticeable in the eyeballs, but as the accumulation progresses, the
entire skin becomes discolored. The urine color may darken.
Jaundice, of course, is not a specific symptom of cirrhosis and

can occur whenever there is overproduction of bile pigments, liver damage of any sort to the point where the organ cannot excrete them, or blockage of the bile ducts.

Just as there are multiple causes of jaundice, so are there many causes of ascites, or the collection of fluid in the abdomen. When it occurs during the course of cirrhosis, it is associated with portal hypertension, that is, a high pressure in the large vein that brings blood from most of the abdominal structures to be circulated through the liver before it returns to the heart. Newly formed regenerative nodules of liver tissue press and distort the branches of the portal vein, increasing the pressure within the system and contributing to the backup of fluid in the abdomen. As much as several gallons of liquid may accumulate in these persons. The spleen also enlarges under these circumstances, and the veins in the esophagus and upper stomach become enlarged. The latter form varicose veins in the esophagus. If these veins break, massive bleeding results, and this is the cause of death in many patients with portal cirrhosis.

When the disease progresses, the victim becomes emaciated and weaker, and hepatic coma may occur. As liver function worsens, the mental changes of impending coma may appear; he becomes confused and drowsy and finally lapses into a stupor and then coma. Many cirrhotic patients die in this manner.

Physical examination of a patient with portal cirrhosis often shows many findings, so that the diagnosis can be suspected on the initial visit to the doctor. The presence of jaundice or abdominal swelling always raises the question of cirrhosis. "Liver spots" are tiny red areas in the skin with delicate red lines emanating from the spot, so that they look like red spiders in the skin. Redness of the palms (like the "spiders," also seen in pregnant women and in other conditions) can occur. The large liver and spleen may be felt on examination. Muscle wasting can be obvious, especially around the front of the shoulders. The testes become soft as a result of certain hormone changes caused by the liver's failure and other metabolic changes of gradual liver destruction.

There are no laboratory tests that are specific for the diagnosis of portal cirrhosis, but the diagnosis can usually be made on the basis of the medical history, physical examination, and blood tests showing interference with liver function. Liver function tests are most useful in following the course of the disease and improve when healing is predominant and become worse as liver damage progresses.

In cases where there is doubt about the diagnosis, a liver biopsy should confirm the diagnosis and provide information about the severity of the process. This involves anesthetizing the skin overlying the liver with an injection through a small needle, then inserting a specially designed larger needle into the liver and withdrawing a tiny piece of liver tissue. The tissue is then examined under the microscope and the actual structural changes can be observed. The entire procedure is brief and involves only a minimal amount of pain. Where there is deep jaundice or where blood clotting is impaired, some danger is involved in liver biopsy, and the procedure may not be possible in the sickest patients.

Although there is no cure for portal cirrhosis, discontinuing the use of alcohol, careful attention to nutrition, and prevention or early treatment of complications will provide a longer and more useful life for patients with this disease. Those who continue to drink alcoholic beverages have a five-year survival rate of 40 percent; that is, of every ten persons with portal cirrhosis who continue to drink after the disease is recognized, only four out of ten will live as long as five years. Of those who stop drinking when the diagnosis is first made, six out of ten will survive for longer than five years. The outlook is worse if liver failure has occurred, as manifested by jaundice or ascites (fluid in the abdomen), and still worse if bleeding from varicose veins in the esophagus has occurred or hepatic coma (mental changes as mentioned above) is present.

The first step in treating portal cirrhosis is the absolute avoidance of drinking any sort of alcohol at all in any amount at all. A nutritious diet is essential for improvement to take place. Ideally, large amounts of proteins should be eaten in order to make up deficits, but this could be harmful if there are signs of impending hepatic coma. These signs consist of confusion, drowsiness or abnormal excitement, a typical slow flapping tremor of the outstretched fingers when the upper extremity is held straight out with the wrists cocked up, and typical brain wave changes. Under these circumstances, protein should be restricted because ammonia and other products of the metabolism of protein will make the hepatic coma worse. Salt should be restricted in the diet when there is any swelling of the abdomen or ankles, and diuretic drugs may be needed to eliminate the fluid. Other measures are available for the treatment of hepatic coma, such as certain antibiotics to remove the intestinal bacteria that form ammonia, correction of the electrolyte imbalance in the blood, which usually accompanies this condition, provision of nitrogen-free food and removal of precipitating causes.

An operation is available for those persons who have developed portal hypertension (see above) as a complication of their portal cirrhosis. This procedure shunts the blood from the portal vein away from the liver and directly into the inferior vena cava and thus to the heart. This sort of by-pass is sometimes done in an emergency for acute bleeding from esophageal veins but is a dangerous procedure because of the universally poor condition of the persons in whom this occurs. The operation is usually successful in preventing recurrent bleeding and also corrects the blood changes that enlargement of the spleen causes, but there are certain late complications of this surgery, and it is not entered into lightly.

As in all other diseases, prevention is better than any available treatment, and avoiding excessive amounts of alcohol is the best preventive measure. Remember, "bon vivant" means good liver, which is something they often don't have!

Disorders of the Rectum and Anus

Disorders of the terminal portion of the digestive tract are extremely common. Although generally medical texts and physicians rank anal problems as minor disorders (especially those physicians who have not suffered personally from an anal fissure or thrombosed hemorrhoids), anything that interferes with normal bowel evacuation because of pain and discomfort is a major nuisance and inconvenience.

Some appreciation of anatomy as well as correct terminology is necessary to understand these disorders. The *anus* is the opening of the lower bowel. The *rectum* itself is the last portion of the large bowel, approximately six inches long, joining the sigmoid colon above and the anus below. The anus is lined by skin and surrounded by two muscle groups called the internal and external sphincter muscles, which keep the anal walls closed; the anal canal is normally closed except when the urge to defecate causes a relaxation of these muscles. Like the skin in the rest of the body, the anus has an abundant nerve supply, which causes disturbances to be appreciated because of pain. On the other hand, the rectum is innervated by nerves of the autonomic nervous system and contains no pain fibers. Stretching or distension of the rectum with feces is appreciated and usually signals the need to find a bathroom for an evacuation. The rectum lies adjacent to many other structures, so a physician can often evaluate the condition of other pelvic organs—the prostate gland in males, and the cervix, uterus, and vagina in females, by rectal examination.

Many diseases in this area involve the anus, including hemorrhoids, fissures, fistula, and abscess formation. Common to these problems is inflammation in the anal tissues caused by contaminated material from the bowel contents. Cancer of the rectum, polyps, rectal itching, and pilonidal cysts are other important diseases.

Hemorrhoids. Hemorrhoids are veins which, because of inflammation, have undergone thinning and dilatation of their walls. They are in many ways similar to varicose veins in the legs but, by their location, they are exposed to trauma from germ-laden bowel movements. Hemorrhoids may originate from veins in the anal canal, *external hemorrhoids*, or arise in the rectum, *internal hemorrhoids*.

Other factors contributing to hemorrhoid development besides infection and inflammation include pregnancy, certain occupations that require prolonged standing or sitting (such as directing traffic or driving a truck), constipation with resulting straining to evacuate feces, and perhaps a hereditary predisposition.

Many persons are aware of small external hemorrhoids which are usually asymptomatic and offer no problems. Internal hemorrhoids may protrude during a bowel movement and then recede. Bleeding can occur, especially from internal hemorrhoids during a bowel movement that irritates the venous wall—either a hard stool or straining to evacuate. Bright red blood may be noticed in the toilet bowl or on the toilet tissue. A sudden severe pain may occur in a thrombosed external hemorrhoid (one that has clotted blood in it).

Prevention of symptomatic hemorrhoids depends largely on good anal hygiene. Infection and inflammation predispose to hemorrhoid formation and subsequent thrombosis with acute flare-ups. Unfortunately, many of us, especially men, prefer the ease of showers and seldom, if ever, take a bath. Persons with hemorrhoids should take baths periodically to ensure good anal hygiene, and regularly when the hemorrhoids cause distress. Efforts to regulate bowel movements and maintain soft stools by adequate liquid intake are important. At times, stool softeners are useful.

Symptomatic hemorrhoids, either bleeding or painful, that do not respond to conservative measures require surgical intervention.

The first conservative measures include stool softeners and Sitz baths. Inflammation is often relieved by sitting in hot tubs of water several times a day. Many people with hemorrhoids report relief of symptoms by using any of a number of hemorrhoidal preparations on the market, usually salves and ointments or suppositories. These agents are usually astringents (cause swollen tissue to shrink and decrease in size) or anesthetic agents, which numb the swollen area and cut down on pain.

Usually, surgery for hemorrhoids includes hospitalization with excision of the diseased hemorrhoids under local anesthesia. Best results are achieved when the procedure is performed by a skilled general surgeon or a proctologist, a specialist in anal-rectal disorders. A recent surgical technique, tying of the hemorrhoid(s) with an elastic band, which is followed by sloughing of the hemorrhoid, appears to yield good results and can be done as an office procedure.

In evaluating anal bleeding, certainly in patients above the age of 35 years, the presence of hemorrhoids should not lull the physician into accepting them as the source of the bleeding. A thorough examination by means of a proctosigmoidoscope should be performed to rule out polyps or rectal cancer.

Anal Fissure.   An anal fissure is an ulcer of the anal skin caused by infection and poor anal hygiene. The fissure itself appears as a linear crack in the anal wall.

Anal fissures may be extremely painful. The pain that is produced by defecation is caused by spasm or tightening of the anal sphincter inside and can last several minutes or longer. Because this pain comes to be associated with a bowel movement, constipation usually develops.

Temporary relief of pain is achieved by using hot compresses, tub baths, or anesthetic ointments to numb the painful areas. Permanent relief requires surgical removal and excision of the entire fissure and surrounding tissue.

Anal Fistula and Abscess.   Anal fistula is caused by an infectious process beginning in an *anal crypt*, a glandular cavity located in the anal canal. The fistula is actually the opening in the anal crypt and a tunnel or passage made by the infectious process burrowing through the anal wall in various directions to resurface at secondary openings in the tissues around the anus. Localized collections of pus, called abscesses, may form.

Pain in the anal area is the chief symptom of an anal fistula or abscess. The pain may be relieved by spontaneous drainage of the pus through a secondary opening. Surgical intervention with opening up of the entire fistula tract by an experienced surgeon can cure this problem.

Pilonidal Cyst. Difficulties in the region of the lower spine are often due to a *pilonidal cyst*. Patients sometimes refer erroneously to this area as their tailbone, implying an ancestral origin from primitive man-like creatures.

A pilonidal cyst is a birth defect occurring in the area of the tip of the spine, the sacrococcygeal region. The cyst lining or cavity is epithelium that was originally destined to form skin but that develops instead under the skin of the lower spine in or near the midline. The pilonidal cyst communicates via small channels or sinuses with openings in the skin in the center of the lower spine. Often, tufts of hair arise from these cysts, hence their designation, pilonidal, which means nest of hair.

Through these openings in the skin, bacterial contamination and infection may occur. Infection of pilonidal cysts is often caused by trauma; for example, in military personnel it could follow a hard, bumpy ride in a jeep.

The symptoms of an infected pilonidal cyst are similar to infection in any other region—pain and swelling. The cyst may drain spontaneously, and often chronic draining sinus tracts are present.

Treatment is surgical and consists of opening the various sinuses into the cyst, excising overhanging margins of skin and allowing the wound to heal.

Rectal Itching. Doctors use the term *pruritis ani* for rectal itching. At times, the condition is a serious disturbance with the affected area of skin thickened, macerated, and secondarily infected because of the patient's constant and vigorous scratching in an effort to relieve the intolerable itching. Most often, rectal itching is a mild nuisance and social embarrassment. The causes are numerous, including local as well as psychogenic causes.

Poor anal hygiene with infrequent bathing can cause rectal

itching. Sweating and the contact of underclothes on the skin around the rectum can produce discomfort; strong detergents or bleaches used in washing undergarments may irritate sensitive skin and cause itching in already inflamed skin.

Any rectal problem associated with excess moisture or discharge irritates the skin and may lead to pruritis ani—anal fissures, sinus tracts and fistulas, hemorrhoids, certain forms of venereal disease, or anal warts. Pinworms, a parasitic infection, are associated with rectal itching, especially occurring and awakening the sufferer in the middle of the night, when the worm migrates to the outside from the rectum to deposit its eggs.

Not uncommonly, no local cause for rectal itching can be found and the condition represents a nervous habit or compulsion.

Treatment depends on successfully identifying the possible local factors and correcting them. Improved local hygiene provided by bathing and using mild soaps as well as avoidance of strong bleaches and detergents on underwear can solve the problem. Local causes, such as hemorrhoids or anal fissures, respond to appropriate treatment. A search for the eggs of the pinworm, if successful, allows for eradication of the infection by medication. Very often, other members of the family harbor the worms because of sharing bedding and toilet facilities.

When no specific cause of itching is found, temporary relief may be achieved from antihistamine drugs. Salves or creams containing steroids and drug combinations reduce inflammation and itching. Tranquilizers are effective in relieving itching associated with nervous tension.

Hernias

Hernias are of several types and may be located on the outside of the body where they can be seen or felt, or inside the body. They are named according to their location.

External hernias may be located in the groin area and are called *inguinal hernias*, under an incision site, *incisional hernia*, in the area of the navel, *umbilical hernia*, or below the groin in the upper thigh, *femoral hernia*. An example of an internal hernia is a *hiatus hernia*.

Inguinal Hernia. Inguinal hernias or ruptures are very common and usually occur in males. They can be located on either side of the groin, right or left, or be present on both sides. They are caused by a weakness or defect in the lower abdominal wall producing a hole or potential passage for a loop of bowel. The human testes arise in the flank area contiguous to the kidneys and descend during the development of the fetus finally to pass through the abdominal wall to settle in the scrotum. This descent leaves a potential weakness for a hernia to develop. Many hernias are present at birth and are detected at an early age.

Hernias can develop at any age. Heavy activity and lifting put a strain on the abdominal muscles and can allow for the development of a rupture or hole through which a loop of bowel or fat may protrude.

Persons with chronic constipation who have to strain to have a bowel movement may develop a hernia because of an increase in abdominal pressure. Smokers who cough frequently may eventually weaken the abdominal wall and form a hernia. Older men who have enlargement of the prostate gland may have difficulty in urinating and are prone to develop an inguinal hernia.

The hernia, which is actually a mass of tissue, usually a loop of bowel, or a piece of omental fat or bladder wall, may be quite small or as large as a grapefruit.

Many times a person becomes aware of a hernia when he discovers a lump in his groin. He may have been doing some strenuous lifting and have felt some discomfort in his groin. Often a hernia is completely asymptomatic and is discovered during an insurance examination or a routine physical examination.

A hernia will protrude when the person stands or when he coughs and raises the intra-abdominal pressure. When he lies down, the hernia often disappears into the abdomen or can be pushed back. This type of hernia is known as a *reducible hernia*. If the hernia cannot be reduced back into the abdomen, it is trapped and is called an *incarcerated hernia*. The incarcerated hernia, a loop of bowel protruding through an opening in the wall of the abdomen, may become swollen and inflamed by the pressure on it, and the circulation to that portion of the bowel may be reduced, producing a *strangulated hernia*.

Hernias should be repaired. A repair of a reducible hernia or incarcerated hernia carries a negligible risk; whereas a strangulated hernia may have significant complications and may even lead to death. Having an inguinal hernia is like walking around with a stick of dynamite in the back pocket. Nothing may ever happen, or the dynamite can explode tonight.

Many older men have had hernias for years and have escaped problems. Some wear a truss, or a belt with a metal plate that applies pressure over the weak area of the abdominal wall.

A hernia repair done by a skilled surgeon is generally successful. The defect is repaired so that no weakness remains in the tissues of the abdominal wall. Occasionally, despite surgery, the area breaks down again and a hernia develops again. Generally, elective surgery involves a four or five day hospital stay. Postoperatively, a convalescence of approximately one month at home is advised, and no heavy manual work is allowed for at least three months.

Incisional Hernia. A hernia can develop at the incision site following any abdominal operation. Abdominal surgery involves cutting through and dissecting many different muscle layers. At times the repair of the various muscle layers is inadequate, or the muscles are so weakened that a strong repair is not done or is not possible. Under these circumstances, a defect develops that allows for the protrusion of abdominal contents through the incision site, especially noted when standing. Just as in the case of an inguinal hernia, the hernia may become incarcerated or strangulated, so that surgical repair is recommended when possible to restore the weak portion of the abdominal wall.

Umbilical Hernia. In the uterus, the fetus is nourished by the umbilical cord, which allows for the transport of oxygen and nourishment to the fetus and the removal of waste products. This exchange occurs by the attachment of the umbilical cord to the placenta and maternal circulation, and connects internally to the fetal circulation. Although the umbilical cord is cut at birth when the child breathes on his own, the passage of the cord through the umbilical opening or navel leaves a potential muscle weakness that may serve for the eventual development of an umbilical hernia. The factors previously cited that may precipitate the occurrence of inguinal or incisional hernias apply here as well.

Of interest is the high occurrence of umbilical hernias in black infant males, most of which do not require surgery but improve with time.

Hiatal Hernia. A hiatal hernia is internal and, therefore, is not diagnosed by feeling an abnormal lump. A hiatal hernia refers to the protrusion of part of the stomach through an opening in the diaphragm, a muscle that separates the chest, lungs, and heart from the abdominal cavity. Hiatal hernias are also known as diaphragmatic hernias. At times, a hiatal hernia is massive, with the bulk of the stomach located in the chest and behind the heart. Normally, the diaphragm helps maintain the integrity of the gate mechanism or sphincter that allows for the passage of food and liquids into the stomach but prevents the regurgitation of acid into the esophagus. When a hiatal hernia is present, acid can now regurgitate and cause heartburn.

The symptoms of indigestion and heartburn usually cause the person to seek medical attention, and an evaluation of the stomach by an upper gastrointestinal series demonstrates the presence of a hiatal hernia. Since hiatal hernias are located behind the heart, symptoms of hiatal hernia may mimic those of cardiac disease. The symptoms of a hiatal hernia generally are aggravated by foods that stimulate acid production—spicy foods, alcohol, coffee, etc. The symptoms are worse when the person eats and lies down, further allowing reflux or regurgitation of acid.

Treatment of a hiatal hernia is generally by medical means. A bland diet is recommended and antacids used after eating to neutralize acid. Persons are advised not to eat before going to bed or not to lie down following meals. At times, reflux of acid contents into the esophagus and mouth can be prevented by elevating the head of the bed with six-inch blocks. In a small number of cases surgery may have to be performed when symptoms cannot be adequately controlled medically. Persistent regurgitation of acid into the esophagus produces a chemical irritation leading to inflammation and scarring and narrowing of the esophagus. Massive bleeding can occur and require surgery.

Symptoms you should know about:

Vomiting blood. Whenever blood is vomited, it is an emergency and the doctor should be seen immediately. Partly digested blood may appear dark brown like coffee grounds.

Black ("tarry") stools. Unless iron-containing medication is being taken, black stools should be considered an emergency condition.

Fresh rectal bleeding. The passage of bright red blood

during or after a bowel movement should always be investigated for its cause, but it is usually not an emergency.

Constipation and diarrhea.   A change in bowel habits lasting more than two weeks ought to be discussed with the doctor.

Abdominal pain.   Pain in the abdomen has many causes, as dealt with in this chapter.

Jaundice.   The first sign of jaundice is usually a yellow color in the eyes. Later the skin becomes yellow. Sometimes very dark-colored urine and light-colored (like clay) stools accompany jaundice. This always requires seeing the doctor for diagnosis as to the cause and treatment.

THE URINARY SYSTEM

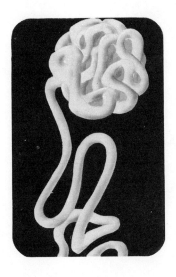

Normal Kidney Function

Let us suppose that a design engineer was given the task of developing an efficient system of waste disposal of the potentially poisonous byproducts formed during the otherwise useful chemical processes of the body's metabolism. In addition, the liquid medium (blood) transporting the waste materials must be reusable and is vital for normal function (health), and contains many important constituents that have to be salvaged and recycled. If he were talented enough, he would produce a machine that was an artificial kidney.

Fortunately for us, we have two kidneys, a fraction of the size of an artificial one, located in the flank area—one on the right side and the other on the left side. (See illustration 6.) If one of the kidneys is damaged or diseased and removed, the remaining kidney, if otherwise normal, can function perfectly well to maintain normal health.

The kidneys, which account for less than one percent of our body weight, receive 25 to 30 percent of the total body blood flow each minute, and through an elaborate filtering system remove many substances from the blood.

Each kidney contains approximately one million separate filtering units called nephrons. The individual nephron contains a filtering network of tiny blood vessels called capil-

The Urinary System

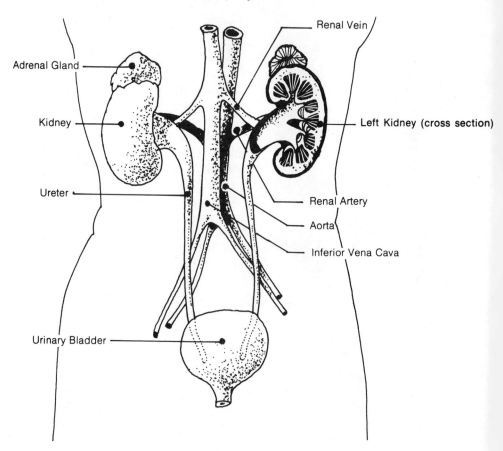

Illustration 6

laries in a basket-like arrangement known as a glomerulus. From the glomerulus, a winding loop or channel lined by kidney cells known as tubular cells modifies the fluid filtered by the glomerulus, which then drains into the collecting system of each kidney and into the ureter to the bladder.

As the fluid filtered by the glomerulus flows by various segments of the tubular cell lined loop, some substances are entirely removed and reabsorbed to re-enter the blood and circulation. Other substances are partially reabsorbed and retained, and some are secreted or added to the fluid depending on the needs of the body. The final volume of fluid produced depends on the body's need to preserve or get rid of water and is under the hormonal control of a protein secreted by the pituitary gland of the brain called the anti-diuretic hormone (ADH). Consuming large amounts of fluid or alcohol leads to copious amounts of urine production, since ADH release is shut off. If a person is dehydrated and thirsty, ADH is produced and maximal water reabsorption occurs in the kidney leading to small amounts of concentrated urine.

Normally, each minute 125 cc. of plasma is filtered by the glomeruli, or 170 liters per day! The final volume of fluid or urine excreted per day averages but 1 or 2 liters. The net result of the filtering, reabsorption, and secretion by the various components of the nephron is the removal of many waste products of the body metabolism, including nitrogen products such as urea, and various acids; the conservation of many important minerals and salts (calcium, phosphorus, sodium, chloride, potassium); the maintenance of a normal body acid content; and preservation of plasma volume by means of water conservation or loss as described above.

In addition to their function in conservation of vital body salts, maintenance of plasma volume, and elimination of waste products, the kidneys have been recognized in recent years as the site of production of important chemical mediators or hormones. Blood pressure and sodium control is directly influenced by a hormone produced in the kidney, called renin, which responds to changes in bloodflow through the kidney. Erythropoietin formed in the kidneys influences the production of red blood cells by the bone marrow tissue. The kidney also influences the absorption of calcium from the gastrointestinal tract by converting vitamin D to a more active and potent form.

The Kidney in Disease

Any disease process that damages or injures the kidneys causes an alteration of renal function that may be either minimal or so severe that life is not possible without alternative measures, such as use of an artificial kidney, called dialysis, or transplant of a kidney from a compatible donor.

When renal function is disturbed, a series of events occurs that reflect malfunction of the various parts of the nephron. Toxic products are not properly eliminated and accumulate in the blood, and vital salts and chemical constituents of the body are not conserved. These abnormalities are easily detected by various blood tests that measure the levels of these substances. Kidney failure or uremia (the retention of urea) refers to the clinical picture and laboratory findings produced by these events and is the final expression of many different kidney disorders.

The kidneys may be seriously damaged by any process causing hypotension or shock. This can occur from serious trauma in an accident with significant hemorrhage, or in circulatory collapse caused by a serious infection. Kidney damage may result from any process in the lower urinary tract, including the bladder, prostate, or ureters, which blocks urine flow and prevents adequate drainage or runoff from a kidney or kidneys. This type of obstruction causes a build up of pressure above the blocked area and distension, ultimately damaging the kidneys.

Very often kidney failure is the result of a disease process that damages the kidney itself. The kidney may be the primary site of a disease process or may be secondarily involved by numerous disorders that affect many parts of the body—a systemic disease. But because normal kidney function is so vital for good health, the manifestations of kidney disease may be the most serious component of an otherwise generalized process.

Examples of generalized or systemic diseases that may cause major renal failure include hypertension, diabetes mellitus, and connective tissue disorders.

The kidney is often damaged in hypertension, a disorder that injures the blood vessels, arteries, and arterioles, causing a process termed nephrosclerosis, with various degrees of renal failure.

Several types of kidney disease commonly occur in diabetes mellitus, including serious damage to the glomeruli called glomerulosclerosis. Among juvenile diabetics, whose disease begins before age fifteen years, renal failure is a leading cause of death.

Connective tissue diseases, such as lupus erythematosus, are associated with circulating immune complexes, which are antibodies combined with antigens that are often trapped in the glomerulus, causing damage to the capillary bed. Kidney disease and renal failure may be the prominent feature of this disease, although many other organs can be involved.

Many other illnesses not primarily involving the kidneys may cause kidney damage and failure, including multiple myeloma, sickle cell disease, and gout, to cite just a few.

Primary Kidney Diseases

The kidneys can be the chief site of a disease process. Various kidney disorders generally involve specific sites of the structural unit of the kidney—the nephron. A disease may affect the *glomerulus, or the proximal* or *distal tubules,* sections of the channel lined by specialized cells that modify and alter the composition of the fluid filtered initially by the glomerulus.

There are several uncommon congenital defects that can interfere with the normal function of a portion of the nephron. Certain chemicals, if ingested, usually accidentally, can cause serious kidney damage, including carbon tetrachloride and ethylene glycol (antifreeze fluid). Several important kidney diseases comprise most primary kidney problems and are dealt with below, including glomerulonephritis, pyelonephritis, and analgesic abuse. Kidney stones, which can develop because of abnormalities in calcium and uric acid metabolism, will also be discussed in this section. Ultimately, any kidney disorder that produces sufficient kidney damage leading to renal failure will affect the entire body. The generalized chemical disturbances of kidney failure alter the functioning of the heart, gastrointestinal tract, peripheral nerves, and blood-forming tissues.

Glomerulonephritis. The term nephritis means inflammation of the kidneys, and glomerulonephritis refers to the glomeruli as the site of the inflammatory process. Although glomerulonephritis can be suspected on clinical grounds and by laboratory tests, the diagnosis is firmly established by a pathologist examining kidney tissue obtained from a kidney biopsy (removal of a core of kidney tissue using a special cutting needle). Microscopic examination, often with a special microscope called an electron microscope, which allows study of minute portions of the cell structure, enables the pathologist to identify hallmarks of this illness. Glomerulonephritis is divided into acute and chronic forms, on the basis of differences in cause and the course of the disease. Since any tissue has a limited number of responses to injury, other disorders can produce changes in the glomeruli that are indistinguishable from glomerulonephritis by routine microscopic findings. Bacterial endocarditis and systemic lupus erythematosus can cause a form of glomerulonephritis, but other features of these diseases distinguish them from classical acute and chronic glomerulonephritis.

Acute glomerulonephritis is much more common in children and young adults and seldom occurs in older people. The disorder commonly follows an infection with Group A Streptococcus, especially with certain strains. The disease does not involve infection of the kidney by the streptococcus organism and develops one to four weeks after the infection, which is usually a pharyngitis ("strep" throat), but it can occur after a streptococcal skin infection. The delay from the initial infection to the onset of the kidney disease suggests some type of allergic or hypersensitivity reaction to the streptococcal germ. Although experimental studies tend to support this conclusion, not all cases of acute glomerulonephritis can be related to a previous streptococcal infection, and other bacteria and viruses have been implicated in causing the disease. At times, no history of any preceding infection is available.

The patient usually seeks medical attention because of bloody urine. In addition, depending on the degree of kidney involvement, various other symptoms are noted. Complaints include swelling around the eyes, loss of appetite, nausea, vomiting, malaise, and headaches. In cases with significant hypertension, heart failure and convulsions may develop.

Examination of the urine, called a urinalysis, points to inflammation in the glomeruli. Protein is detected, as well as red blood cells and red blood cell casts.

The diagnosis of acute glomerulonephritis following a streptococcal infection is not difficult, especially with a history of a recent sore throat caused by Group A Streptococcus or blood tests that show a rising level of antibodies against streptococcus, together with typical findings in the urine.

There is no effective treatment for acute glomerulonephritis. The complications of hypertension and congestive heart failure require treatment. The majority of patients with this disease, certainly 90 to 95 percent of children, have complete healing of the glomeruli, although red blood cells in the urine may persist for a few months. Kidney function remains normal. If serial biopsies of the kidneys show that healing of the glomeruli has not occurred and active disease, with progressive inflammatory changes, scarring, and damage is noted, the patient will go on to develop chronic glomerulonephritis with various degrees of kidney failure.

Most patients with chronic glomerulonephritis are unable to report having any preceding illness similar to acute glomerulonephritis. Often the disease develops insidiously without any known inciting factor. Many patients have no symptoms at all when the condition is first suspected. The patient may be found to have hypertension with blood tests showing kidney dysfunction. A routine urinalysis may show the presence of protein as the first evidence of kidney disease.

In chronic glomerulonephritis, examination of the urine reveals, in addition to the protein leakage which is a constant feature, the presence of various types of casts composed of protein and cellular debris formed in the kidney tubules. As the disease progresses, inability of the kidney to concentrate the urine and conserve water also develops. Besides the abnormal findings on urinalysis, various blood tests of kidney function and salt (electrolyte) concentration become abnormal. X-rays of the kidneys generally show both kidneys to be smaller than normal. A kidney biopsy usually reveals evidence of chronic glomerulonephritis.

Patients with chronic glomerulonephritis can be followed for many years and be relatively asymptomatic before definite signs of kidney failure appear. As a rough rule, few symptoms of chronic renal failure develop until renal function deteriorates to below 20 percent of normal. An occasional patient may seek medical attention when symptoms of far advanced renal failure have developed, including nausea, vomiting, weakness, and fatigue. At this point, hypertension and heart failure may be present and marked abnormalities of kidney function may be detected, including uremia, acidosis, and electrolyte imbalances. Death usually occurs as renal function is no longer sufficient to sustain life, unless a program of kidney dialysis is begun, with a possible goal of eventually receiving a kidney transplant.

About half the patients with chronic glomerulonephritis develop the nephrotic syndrome, consisting of massive loss of protein in the urine, hypoalbuminemia (very low levels of the protein albumin, in the blood), increased levels of cholesterol in the blood, and extensive fluid retention in the body. The nephrotic syndrome usually takes place after several years of chronic glomerulonephritis, but it may be the initial evidence of the disease. It lasts for months to a few years, and during this time renal function usually deteriorates.

Pyelonephritis. The term "kidney infection" is used quite generally for any infection that may be located in the kidneys or the urinary tract, which includes the urethra (the tube bringing the urine from the bladder to the outside) and the bladder (the reservoir of urine). Pyelonephritis refers to bacterial infection of the kidneys, and is divided into the *acute* bacterial infection with symptoms of urinary tract infection and *chronic pyelonephritis*, which, up until recently, had been considered to result from the cumulative injury to the kidney(s) from previous episodes of acute pyelonephritis. However, most patients, including those who have had multiple attacks of acute pyelonephritis, never progress to chronic pyelonephritis, and the majority of patients who are diagnosed as having chronic pyelonephritis cannot relate a history of having had acute pyelonephritis. Considerable doubt exists regarding the relationship of acute pyelonephritis to chronic pyelonephritis, which is now more often called chronic interstitial nephritis.

Acute pyelonephritis occurs most commonly in females, especially during infancy and the childbearing years. Although acute pyelonephritis can be induced experimentally in animals by seeding the blood with bacteria, most evidence supports the view that infections originate retrograde, namely, from the ascent of bacteria from the urethra and bladder into the kidneys.

Although about one half of patients with acute pyelonephritis have no known cause, in the remaining cases, a predisposing factor can be identified. Any process that obstructs the flow of urine from the kidneys increases the incidence of infection. A prime example is a kidney stone. Females have a short urethra, the distance from the outside, unsterile environment to the sterile bladder, being about one inch. Both female infants (perhaps due to fecal staining) and adult women (perhaps because of urethral trauma caused by sexual relations) have a greater risk of acute pyelonephritis. Patients who undergo any type of urinary tract procedure in which instruments are used, such as the passage of a catheter into the bladder during delivery, or who require cystoscopy, an evaluation of the inside of the urinary bladder, are liable to develop a kidney infection because bacteria gain entrance into the bladder and may ascend to the kidneys. Certain neurological disturbances (multiple sclerosis, poliomyelitis, spinal cord injury) that secondarily interfere with bladder function may require frequent or constant catheterization of the bladder, and repeated urinary tract infections are common. Other disorders associated with acute pyelonephritis include pregnancy itself, sickle cell trait, and diabetes mellitus.

Typical and classic acute pyelonephritis is generally first seen with high fever, a temperature of 101 to 104° F., chills, flank pain, and discomfort on urination. On examining the patient, the doctor may note tenderness over one or both flank areas.

At times, few if any symptoms of this disorder are present, and it may be suspected only by the finding of many pus cells in the urine and a positive urine culture. Burning and discomfort on urination and the finding of increased white blood cells in the urine with a positive urine culture do not allow for distinguishing between a bladder infection and a kidney infection.

Patients with uncomplicated acute pyelonephritis have otherwise normal renal function and normal blood pressure. Those with acute kidney infection in association with obstruction or an anatomical abnormality may have renal damage and abnormal kidney function.

Most cases of acute kidney infection respond well to treatment with an appropriate antibiotic. If a predisposing factor is present and not corrected, repeated infections are the rule, usually caused by the same strain of bacteria, which often develop resistance to the antibiotic previously given in an attempt to eradicate the infection.

The pathologist who examines kidney tissue obtained either at autopsy or during life from a kidney biopsy makes the diagnosis of chronic pyelonephritis based on certain microscopic features, including widespread scarring of the kidney. Many types of injury to the kidney besides infections can lead to these changes, which are termed chronic pyelonephritis. In fact, recent investigation has shown that bacterial infections alone seldom, if ever, cause chronic pyelonephritis, but additional causes are necessary, among them vascular disease (often associated with hypertension), anatomic abnormalities, overuse of analgesic agents (pain medication including phenacetin, aspirin, and acetaminophen), increased levels of uric acid (hyperuricemia), and kidney stones.

Patients with chronic pyelonephritis most often have no symptoms until sufficient renal damage develops to produce the symptoms previously described with uremia and renal failure due to chronic glomerulonephritis. If infection is proved, the use of appropriate antibiotics may improve or stabilize renal function to levels consistent with a relatively normal existence. Often the course of chronic pyelonephritis is compatible with a long survival, as renal failure progresses quite slowly. Hypertension is common in this disorder and may cause congestive heart failure or a stroke unless adequately treated.

Patients with far advanced or end stage renal failure secondary to chronic pyelonephritis require kidney dialysis to maintain life and eventually may be candidates for a kidney transplant.

Kidney Stones.   Kidney stones, or renal calculi, develop quite frequently in otherwise healthy persons. They may develop only once in a lifetime or form repeatedly, with episodes of acute renal pain or colic associated with the passage of the stone from the kidney pelvis, through the ureter into the bladder, and, finally, out through the urethra.

In a typical case, a patient calls the doctor complaining of a severe and excruciating pain which has gradually developed in the previous hour. The discomfort is first located along his flank and is then present in the front of the abdomen and radiating toward the groin. He is admitted to the hospital, given pain medication, and a urine specimen is noted to be bloody. An x-ray film of the abdomen called a KUB shows a suspicious, tiny density along one side of the abdomen and an x-ray of the kidneys obtained by injecting a radiopaque dye (an intravenous pyelogram), shows a stone lodged midway along the course of the ureter with some dilatation of the kidney collecting system (pelvis) above the stone. The patient is encouraged to drink lots of fluid, and later on that day experiences a second bout of severe pain very similar to the initial attack. Further pain medication is given, and shortly thereafter, a stone is passed in his urine, which is recovered by straining the urine specimen. A repeat x-ray taken a few days later shows the previous shadow has disappeared, indicating that the stone has indeed been passed and there no longer is any dilatation of the kidney above the site of obstruction. Analysis of the stone chemically shows it to be made up of calcium oxalate.

It is not entirely clear in most cases why kidney stones form. Racial, dietary, and climatic factors account for some instances of stone formation. Usually, stone formation requires two components, an organic matrix of proteinaceous material (called a nidus) and the crystals that precipitate from urine onto the nidus and constitute the bulk of the stone. In normal urine, despite a high concentration of crystalloid substances (calcium, phosphates, oxalates, uric acid) in solution, a favorable balance of other constituents are present to prevent crystal formation. Kidney stones not uncommonly develop in the setting of a kidney infection that promotes the presence of proteinaceous material or nidus for crystals to deposit. Infection of urine by urea-splitting bacteria alters the solubility of crystalloids by changing the urine acidity, favoring stone formation.

Calcium stones, the most commonly encountered ones, may develop in patients who excrete excess amounts of calcium in the urine. In most cases, no cause or underlying disease can be identified, although a family history of kidney stones may be present. In hyperparathyroidism, a disorder characterized almost always by a benign tumor of a parathyroid gland, excess parathyroid hormone causes bone reabsorption and release of calcium, raising the blood and urine levels of calcium. Kidney stones develop in 20 percent of such cases, and hyperparathyroidism accounts for perhaps 5 percent of all calcium stones.

Uric acid stones develop in conditions associated with high levels of blood uric acid and increased excretion of uric acid in the urine. Gout, acute attacks of arthritis in one joint caused by uric acid crystals, is often associated with uric acid kidney stones. Several other uncommon disorders, such as cystinuria, can cause stones.

The ideal approach in a person who has a kidney stone involves collection of the stone when it is passed and analysis to identify the constituents of the stone. If a urinary tract infection is present, cultures of the urine with identification of the bacterial agent and treatment with an appropriate antibiotic is undertaken. Urinary tract infections predispose to stone formation, and stones, by interfering with adequate urine flow and drainage, are often associated with infection. The need to perform urological surgery to remove a stone also predisposes to the risk of introducing infection. An anatomical abnormality identified by an intravenous pyelogram (x-ray of the kidney and urinary tract) that is associated with repeated urinary tract infections and kidney stones may require surgical intervention and attempted repair. Blood studies are usually done to help in ruling out disturbances of calcium and uric acid metabolism. If hyperparathyroidism is proved, surgical exploration of the neck and removal of the involved gland(s) is necessary. Excess uric acid levels in the blood with secondary increased uric acid excretion in the urine can be controlled by certain drugs.

Surgery may be required to remove large stones in the kidney or ones that lodge in the ureter, are not passed, and are associated with renal colic and obstruction to urine flow from the involved kidney.

Patients who form stones are encouraged to drink large amounts of fluids so that they will excrete lots of urine (over a quart per day) in order to help maintain crystals in solution.

Kidney Dialysis

Dialysis refers to the exchange of molecules of substances (solutes) from one fluid to another by diffusion through a semipermeable membrane. A simple example would be a chamber containing salt water on one side and pure or distilled water on the other. If the membrane or lining separating the two fluids were permeable, or porous, to the molecules of sodium and chloride (salt), these would diffuse from the salt water chamber to the distilled water until the concentrations were the same on both sides of the membrane.

Hemodialysis is the process when blood from an artery of a patient with chronic renal failure (uremia) containing high levels of urea, creatinine, uric acid, sulfates, phosphates, and various other substances is circulated through an artificial kidney on one side of a membrane, while a balanced or physiological solution circulates on the other side. Over a period of time, the high concentrations of "toxic substances" in the blood are reduced as they diffuse into the fluid of the dialysis bath.

Patients may undergo dialysis for acute reversible kidney damage, where one to three weeks is needed for repair and restoration of renal function. Examples of this type of problem include acute shock from blood loss or from overwhelming infection, or from certain drugs that have damaged the kidneys. Dialysis may also be used for patients with acute poisoning caused by potentially lethal doses of barbiturates or other sedatives.

For end stage renal disease with severe kidney failure, patients undergo dialysis on a long-term basis. To facilitate the procedure, artificial shunts are created in the arm between an artery and vein in order to keep the blood vessel open. A plastic tube in the artery removes the blood from the patient and carries it to the dialysis unit, and another plastic tube then returns the blood to the vein. Patients usually require two or three sessions per week of several hours each in order to reverse and control the symptoms of uremia and chronic renal failure. Some patients with otherwise terminal renal failure have been kept alive for several years while efforts to find a suitable kidney donor for a kidney transplant have gone on. Needless to say, the financial burden of such dialysis is a major problem. In addition, the need for frequent interruptions of normal living for the vital dialyses imposes an emotional strain on the patient and his family.

Organ Transplants

The ability to transplant a normal organ from a donor to a recipient with end stage disease and restore normal function and improved health must rank as one of the greatest scientific accomplishments of the current century.

Heart transplants had been attempted in 202 patients through 1972, with 29 patients surviving more than two years, and 6 patients living beyond four years. Improving results have recently been reported from Stanford University where 153 heart transplants had been performed before September 1978, with 64 survivors into 1979, one of whom was living more than 8 years after surgery. Bone marrow transplants are currently being carried out in a few medical centers for acute leukemia, deficiency of the immune system or bone marrow failure. Of 182 liver transplants done as of 1972, only 3 patients survived beyond three years. Lung transplants done in 32 patients during the last ten years have been quite disappointing, with only 3 patients living for more than thirty days with a functioning graft. Recent efforts to transplant the pancreas also have been generally unsuccessful.

The greatest success rate and largest experience with organ transplants have been in kidney transplants, either from a living donor or a cadaver kidney, one obtained from a patient with normal kidneys immediately upon death. The highest success rate is from a relative of the patient who shares similar antigenic traits known as histocompatibility genes. Approximately 75 percent of organ grafts (transplants) from a blood relative survive and function for at least a year and around 50 percent of cadaver kidneys do as well in the recipient. Patients with functioning grafts have an average survival of around two and a half years, and those living more than five years are not uncommon.

In order to circumvent the normal body's response to foreign tissue (and the body treats a transplanted organ, unless from an identical twin, as different and attempts to destroy it), powerful drugs called immunosuppressants are given. Unfortunately, by modifying and altering the usual bodily defense mechanisms, we expose the recipient of a graft to the risk of unusual infectious diseases and an increased chance of developing a malignant disease.

Lower Urinary Tract Disease

The urinary bladder, which should not be confused with the gallbladder, is a reservoir or chamber that stores the urine from the kidneys. The bladder is quite distensible, like a balloon, and can store up to several hundred cubic centimeters of urine. The bladder is located in the center of the lower abdomen or above the pubic bone, in the suprapubic region. The opening of the bladder, which is located at the bottom or base of the organ, is usually closed by an arrangement of muscle fibers called a sphincter. When the bladder fills through two tubes from the kidneys—the ureters—and distends, the urge to urinate is felt and voluntary relaxation of the bladder sphincter along with contraction of the muscular wall of the bladder initiates urination.

The urethra is the channel from the bladder to the outside. In the female, the urethra is only about an inch long, opening to the outside into the vulva. In the male, the urethral passage is several inches long, the channel passing through the penis to the outside. Bladder infections are much more common in women because of the relatively short urethra or passageway from the bladder to the outside.

Various problems can interfere with normal urination. Obstruction to the outflow tract of the bladder is very common in men because of enlargement of the prostate gland. Injuries to the spinal cord itself secondary to trauma or an accident, or to the nerves that control the bladder, which can occur in diabetes, can prevent proper functioning of the bladder muscle and sphincter. Loss of urinary control or incontinence can be a serious problem or a source of constant embarrassment. Bladder infections and bladder tumors, both benign and malignant, are additional disorders.

Bladder Infections (cystitis). Bladder infections are quite common in females because of ready access of bacteria into the bladder. Young girls should be taught at an early age to cleanse their anal area by wiping from front to back in order to minimize the possibility of introducing bacterial infection. Although infection is usually confined to the bladder, it may spread up the ureters and cause serious kidney infections as well. Bladder infection commonly occurs in newlywed women and is called "honeymoon cystitis." It is recommended that women empty their bladders after having sexual relations and before retiring to bed in order to minimize the possibility of bladder infections.

Symptoms of bladder infection include the urge to urinate frequently, with burning and discomfort and often only small amounts of urine passed. Lower abdominal distress and an uncomfortable pressure sensation are often noted as well as fever.

The urine may be cloudy, or at times, bloody. Examination under the microscope shows white blood cells, often in clumps (pus cells), and bacteria.

Treatment with antibiotics is almost always successful, but recurrences of infection are quite common in some persons. In cases of frequent infections of the lower urinary tract, bladder or urethra, evaluation of the bladder by cystoscopy may be necessary to reveal anatomical abnormalities or reasons for incomplete emptying of the bladder, which predispose to infection. Urine samples collected in as sterile a manner as possible should be obtained to identify the bacteria involved and to determine which antibiotic will be most effective. Fluids are important to maintain a good urine output, which irrigates the bladder and helps to wash out bacteria.

Bladder Tumors. Bladder tumors, either benign growths

called papillomas or malignant ones, are usually discovered when a person seeks medical attention because of an abnormal urine specimen. Blood in the urine, referred to as *hematuria*, is alarming, and warrants investigation to localize the site in the urinary tract as well as the cause of the bleeding. Since bleeding can be coming from the kidneys, ureters, bladder, or urethra, a stepwise evaluation that includes kidney x-rays and cystoscopy is necessary to find the source.

Benign growths are often removed at the time of cystoscopy, but they may recur. Malignant growths require removal of the involved bladder. If the cancer is very superficial and does not penetrate deeply into the bladder wall, and is located in an area of the bladder away from the ureters and outflow tract, a partial excision of the bladder is possible—preserving the rest of the organ. For extensive disease, total removal of the bladder may be necessary, often combined with cobalt radiation prior to or following surgery. If the bladder is removed completely, an artificial bladder is made using a loop of small bowel called an ileal bladder and the ureters are reimplanted into this structure.

Incontinence. Urinary incontinence, or loss of voluntary bladder control, occurs quite frequently, especially in elderly, debilitated, often bedridden patients, who have various chronic diseases. Because bedwetting leads to bedsores, skin ulcers, and serious infections, urinary catheters are often needed to protect the skin. Catheters in this setting are the lesser of two evils, since chronic bladder infection develops when they are used for a long time.

A rather frequent cause of incontinence is seen in women, almost always those who have had multiple pregnancies— *stress incontinence*. This problem develops because repeated stretching of the pelvic tissues during pregnancies causes the bladder to drop, distorting the anatomical relationships of the bladder neck. Uncontrolled wetting, usually initiated by acts such as coughing, laughing, sneezing, or bending can be quite a source of distress. Part of the bladder actually sinks into the vagina and may even protrude, called a cystocele.

Correction of a cystocele and stress incontinence can be achieved if the symptoms are troublesome or severe by surgery to strengthen the loose tissues and restore the proper bladder neck angle.

Cystoscopy. Cystoscopy is a surgical procedure to evaluate urinary tract problems performed by a urologist with the patient under either spinal or local anesthesia. The cystoscope is an instrument introduced via the urethra into the bladder. The urologist can look through one end and study the part of the prostate gland that surrounds the bladder neck and also inspect the interior of the bladder. In addition, the openings, one on either side of the bladder, of the two ureters can be seen. If additional information is needed, catheters can be passed up the ureters into the kidneys, allowing for sampling of urine from either kidney. X-ray visualization of kidney detail following an injection of dye can help to locate and identify tumors or stones in the urinary tract.

Cystoscopy is most commonly performed to evaluate the lower urinary tract, including the urethra, prostate, and bladder; if studies of the kidneys by conventional x-ray have proved unsatisfactory for various reasons, cystoscopy allows their visualization from below through dye introduced into the ureters.

Urinary Catheters. Catheters or tubes made of rubber or silicone may be required to ensure proper emptying and drainage of the bladder. They are used frequently in the case of blockage, which can occur in prostate disease or because of disease in the spinal nerves affecting bladder function (neurogenic bladder). Not uncommonly, temporary use of a catheter is required following surgery due to the combined depressive effects of anesthesia and pain medication on bladder function, as well as the inherent difficulties some people have trying to urinate while lying in bed. Critically ill patients who are unconscious or who require careful monitoring of their fluid intake and output generally require bladder catheters.

Prostate Disorders

The Prostate Gland. The prostate gland is found only in males, but many men become familiar with this part of their anatomy only later in life, when a disorder of the gland causes a problem. This small male accessory sex gland weighs about 20 grams. It contributes part of the secretions that make up the male ejaculate, that is, the fluid that discharges during sexual relations.

The prostate gland surrounds the neck of the urinary bladder and through it passes the urethra—the conduit for passage of urine stored in the bladder. (See illustration 7.) Because of its particular location, disturbances in the prostate gland can

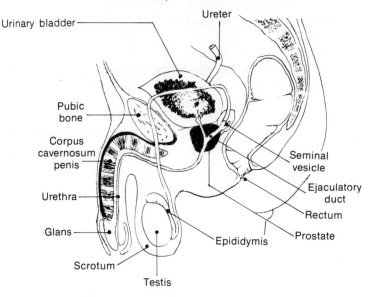

Male Reproductive System:
Side View (sagittal section) of
genital organs and relationship of prostate
to the urinary bladder, urethra, and rectum

Illustration 7

interfere with emptying of the bladder and the ability to urinate. In general, three main disorders can involve the prostate
gland: infection and inflammation, enlargement (or hypertrophy), and cancer.

Inflammation of the Prostate Gland. Prostatitis or
inflammation of the prostate gland may be caused by various
infectious agents, including the bacteria that cause tuberculosis and gonorrhea (a venereal infection), or it may not be
associated with an identifiable agent (nonspecific prostatitis).
Prostatitis may temporarily follow sexual arousal or stimulation not accompanied by ejaculation, due to retained secretions and acute congestion of the gland.

Symptoms of prostatitis include frequent and painful
urination as well as, at times, a discharge from the penis. The
patient may experience aching in the groin or lower back or
rectum. Fever and chills may develop. The disorder must be
distinguished from a kidney or bladder infection or an
infection of the urethra. On rectal examination of a man with

acute prostatitis, the prostate gland is easily felt by the doctor to be lying adjacent to the front wall of the rectum and is noted to be enlarged, boggy, and extremely tender. The urine will contain pus cells and possibly bacteria. A culture obtained from urine, penile discharge, or following massage of the prostate gland itself, allows for identification of the offending bacteria and treatment with the appropriate antibiotic. Pain medications and hot baths also help to relieve discomfort.

Prostatic enlargement.   Benign prostatic hypertrophy refers to enlargement of the prostate gland that ultimately causes difficulties with normal urination. For unknown reasons, the gland enlarges, usually after the age of 50, but perhaps not causing problems until the person is in his 60s or 70s.

The symptoms of obstruction to urine flow caused by enlargement of the prostate are called *prostatism*. The urge to urinate occurs more and more frequently during the day and can awaken the man during his sleep every couple of hours. The size and force of the urine stream diminish, and are often reduced to an intermittent dribble. There may be increasing difficulties initiating urination, with the patient having to wait and strain to produce urine, and following urination, a need to void again quite soon. In the extreme, complete obstruction to the outflow of urine from the bladder causes a build up of back pressure on the ureters and even the kidneys, which can lead to kidney damage or failure, by a process known as hydronephrosis.

Despite urinating with great difficulty, the bladder may not be emptied completely, and may contain a large residual of urine. This pool of urine predisposes to infection, a common complication of prostatism.

The diagnosis of prostate enlargement is easily suspected from the symptoms described above. Additional studies that confirm the diagnosis include an x-ray of the kidney, ureters, and bladder, with a post-voiding film, showing inability to empty the dye from the bladder because of an enlarged prostate. Cystoscopic examination allows for direct visualization of an enlarged gland, encroaching on the bladder floor and urethra, as well as seeing the thickened bladder muscle.

After evaluation by the methods described above, treatment of symptomatic prostatism is surgical. Initially, in some men, temporary catheter drainage is necessary to correct reversible kidney damage. Treatment and control of any bladder infection is also necessary.

The surgical procedure chosen by the urologist depends mainly on the size of the enlarged gland. In the majority of cases the enlarged prostatic tissue can be successfully removed through the urethral opening in the penis by an operation called a transurethral resection. In some cases the prostate enlargement is too great to permit removal this way, and another surgical procedure called a suprapubic prostatectomy is done. This requires a surgical incision in the lower abdomen, opening of the bladder itself, and removing the prostate from above. Both procedures are well tolerated, and a catheter is left in the bladder for a period of time until the tissue has healed and normal urination is possible.

Following prostate surgery, men are usually able to have normal sexual relations except that retrograde ejaculation may occur, that is, the usual fluid containing sperm that is produced at the climax of the male orgasm is ejected back into the bladder and does not flow out through the penis.

Cancer of the prostate.   Cancer of the prostate is one of the most common cancers of men. It rarely occurs in young men and seldom occurs below the age of 50. Its incidence increases with each succeeding decade. Many clinically insignificant, small, and localized tumors are found on careful study of prostatic tissue during a postmortem (autopsy). Fortunately, many of these occult, or hidden, cancers cause no symptoms and can only be detected during life by the pathologist who examines the prostatic tissue removed because of prostatism.

Prostate cancer can first be detected by findings on routine rectal examination. Most cancers develop in the back portion of the gland which lies next to the rectum. The prostate gland can harbor nontender, irregular, hard areas or nodules. Biopsy of any suspicious nodule can establish the diagnosis of prostatic cancer.

Unfortunately, many cases of prostate cancer are detected when the disease is quite advanced, and the patient may have sought medical attention for bone pain due to metastasis, or spread, of the cancer through the blood to the bones—especially to the spine and hip regions.

The only known cure for prostate cancer is complete surgical removal of the gland. This procedure may not be used in some patients because evaluation has shown the disease too advanced and the tumor has spread into bones and adjacent tissues. Measurement of a certain prostatic enzyme in the blood, acid phosphatase, correlates with advanced stages of prostatic cancer.

Even though many patients have extensive disease, palliation, or temporary control, often for years, can be achieved by giving small doses of estrogens (female hormones). Previously, larger doses were used to control the disease, but these now have been associated with increased atherosclerosis and deaths from coronary artery disease. Surgical removal of the testes, called an orchiectomy, also is effective. The male hormones, androgens, apparently promote growth of prostatic cancer.

Good results have also been achieved by injecting radioactive materials into the tumor, causing it to shrink and thus allowing for surgery in an otherwise inoperable prostate. X-ray treatment of involved areas of bone can relieve pain, as can drugs. Chemotherapy, or the use of anticancer drugs, has not been very effective in this disease.

Symptoms you should know about:

Very frequent urination and burning on urination.   These are the cardinal symptoms of a urinary bladder infection.

Bloody urine.   Blood in the urine can be caused by disease in the kidney, ureter, bladder, or urethra, and may be quite serious or only a minor problem. It always requires medical attention.

Backache and **flank pain** may arise in the kidney. **Renal colic,** usually due to the presence of a stone in the ureter, is a severe, crampy pain in the side or abdomen which may be transmitted to the groin or the genitals.

HORMONES AND ENDOCRINE PROBLEMS

6

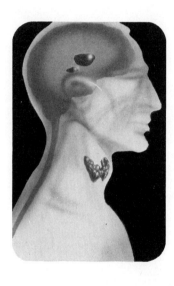

Proper functioning of cellular processes and ultimately tissues and organs of the body requires the actions of various hormones produced by glands located throughout the body. *Hormones* are chemical substances formed in an organ (gland) and delivered into the bloodstream to other parts of the body where they influence basic cellular activities in many important ways. *Endocrinology* is a branch of medicine that deals with the actions of hormones formed by glands both during normal function (physiological) as well as during states of malfunction or disease (pathological). Endocrine or gland disturbances may be due to excess production or underproduction of hormones.

The healthy human body is a wonderful example of a coordinated, integrated machine, made up of complex components serving the various body processes. It has been compared with a symphony orchestra, in which the various sounds and effects (body functions) of the individual instruments and sections of the orchestra (organs) are organized by the conductor (brain) into a harmonious musical rendition (good health).

The Pituitary Gland

The tiny pituitary gland (weighing less than one gram) is the master gland which controls the activities of many endocrine glands, including the thyroid, adrenal, and the sex glands—ovaries and testes. (See illustration 8.)

Disorders of the pituitary develop rather infrequently. Because of its location, pituitary tumors can cause serious brain dysfunction by pressure on adjacent areas. The nerve pathways for vision cross in front of the pituitary and may be affected by pituitary tumors, causing partial blindness. Failure of the pituitary gland to produce its hormones, either partially or completely, leads to secondary failure of the affected target glands.

The anterior pituitary gland produces several hormones. *TSH*, thyroid stimulating hormone, is necessary for the thyroid gland to function normally. *ACTH* (adrenocortico-tropic hormone) is a hormone required for the adrenal gland to produce the crucial hormones known as steroids. *FSH* and *LH*, follicle stimulating hormone and luteinizing hormone respectively, are crucial for the maturation of the sex glands, the testes and especially the ovaries. *Growth Hormone* is necessary for normal human growth; without it, growth fails and dwarfism develops. Too much, produced by pituitary tumors, causes excessive growth—giantism, accounting for the giants who appear in circus sideshows.

The posterior pituitary produces an important hormone called *vasopressin*, which regulates water excretion by the kidney. Failure to produce this hormone causes inability to reabsorb water appropriately by the kidneys, causing the loss of up to 20 liters of water per day. The affected person is constantly thirsty because of his body's failure to conserve water—a disease called *diabetes insipidus*.

It is now felt that cells located within the hypothalamus serve to sense or detect the concentration of various circulating hormones produced by the thyroid, adrenal, and sex glands. When the level of a hormone decreases, chemical mediators produced by the hypothalamus reach the pituitary gland, where the appropriate pituitary hormones are released into the blood and carried to the target. As the target gland (e.g., thyroid gland) responds and increases its production of hormones, the level bathing the hypothalamus increases, leading ultimately to a decrease in the production of stimulatory hormones by the pituitary gland. Thus, a reciprocal relation

The Endocrine System

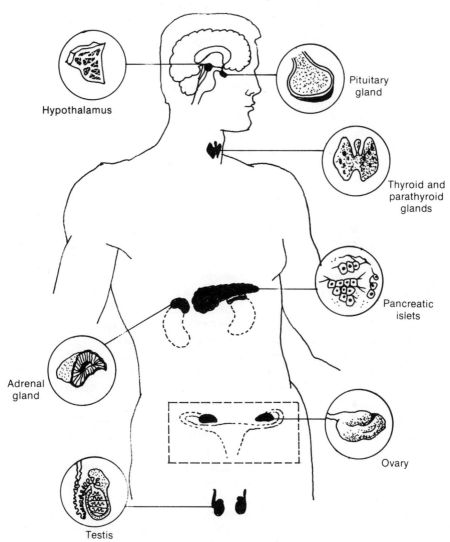

Illustration 8

exists between the pituitary gland and its target glands. An increase in the production of the hormone(s) by the target gland causes a decreased secretion by the pituitary gland, probably mediated by the hypothalamus.

The Thyroid Gland

The thyroid gland is located in the neck, in front of the trachea or windpipe, below and on either side of the thyroid cartilage (Adam's apple). Normally it weighs around 15 to 25 grams. Its chief function is to produce thyroid hormone, which is manufactured from an amino acid called tyrosine and the mineral iodine.

The active thyroid hormones, *thyroxin* and *thyronine*, play a major role in the intracellular energy production that is vital for all tissues. The hormone is important in protein, lipid, carbohydrate, and vitamin A metabolism as well as in normal human growth and maturation of tissues, including muscles, bone, and skin and sexual development.

The thyroid gland performs normally only if the pituitary gland secretes a thyroid stimulating hormone (TSH) that allows the various steps in the manufacture of thyroid hormone to occur. Under the influence of TSH, the thyroid traps and concentrates iodine in the form of organic iodide, synthesizes thyroid hormones in various steps, stores the hormone attached to a large protein within the thyroid gland, and releases the hormone into the bloodstream as needed.

Thyroid disease is by far the commonest disorder of the endocrine glands. Several different disorders of the thyroid gland are possible. These include enlargement of the gland, called a goiter; hyperthyroidism, excess production of thyroid hormone; hypothyroidism, a deficiency of thyroid hormone; tumors, both benign and malignant; and inflammatory diseases.

Goiters. A goiter, an enlargement of the thyroid gland, often quite visible in the neck, can occur with normal or reduced thyroid function (hypothyroidism) called a *nontoxic goiter*, or with hyperthyroidism, a *toxic goiter*.

Nontoxic goiters usually develop because the diet is deficient in iodine. The disease tends to occur in families, especially those living in regions such as the Great Lakes in the United States and mountain areas where iodine is lacking in the water and soil. Iodine normally is derived from water and seafood. When it is lacking, the gland enlarges, often massively, in an effort to secure more iodine.

Other causes, less common, include congenital or birth defects, with absence of one of several enzymes needed in the manufacture or release of thyroid hormones. Chemicals (propylthiouracil) used in treating hyperthyroidism block thyroid hormone production and cause goiters. Other drugs, such as sulfonamides and an antituberculosis drug, para-aminosalicylate (PAS), are weak goitrogens (capable of causing goiter). Certain vegetables contain substances that are weak goitrogens when eaten in large quantities, including rutabaga, kale, cabbage, turnip, peanuts, radishes, and carrots.

Prevention by ensuring adequate iodine in the diet has been achieved to a great extent by adding iodine to salt—iodized salt. Treatment of an established nontoxic goiter with thyroid hormone can be effective in shrinking it. Only rarely is surgery indicated, usually for cosmetic reasons, in removing the goiter.

Hyperthyroidism. Hyperthyroidism is caused by excess production of thyroid hormone. The reasons for this are unknown, but there does appear a relationship to emotional or traumatic events. The disease occurs at any age, commonly at puberty as well as during pregnancy and at the menopause; it seldom occurs in childhood and affects females much more commonly than males.

The thyroid gland is usually diffusely enlarged, and often there is a bulging of the eyeballs called exophthalmos. At times, the condition is associated with a goiter without the accompanying eye changes.

Usually the diagnosis of hyperthyroidism is made without too much difficulty. However, the disorder may be first seen in the elderly as congestive heart failure, and the diagnosis is not suspected because the symptoms and signs are more subtle.

The patient usually has symptoms that include fatigue and weakness (often noted when climbing stairs), increased nervousness, irritability, and insomnia, increased sweating and intolerance to warm weather, rapid and irregular heartbeats (palpitations), weight loss despite a good appetite, and awareness of the protrusion or prominence of the eyeballs, associated with itching and tearing of the eyes.

On examination, the findings suggesting hyperthyroidism include a rapid pulse, warm and moist skin, especially of the hands, fine hair, tremulousness of an outstretched hand (shakes), a visibly enlarged thyroid gland, and a murmur caused by the increased flow of blood through the gland heard with the stethoscope applied over the thyroid gland.

Laboratory confirmation of excess thyroid hormone is obtained by measuring the levels of the hormone in the blood. In pregnancy or in a woman using birth control pills or receiving estrogen hormones, the thyroxin levels may be erroneously elevated because of an increase in the protein that binds thyroxin. Other blood tests measuring the free thyroxin can circumvent this problem.

A radioactive iodine compound can be injected into a person with a suspected overactive thyroid gland and a count made of the radioactivity over the thyroid gland in several hours to 24 hours later. In hyperthyroidism there is a considerably greater concentration and hence percentage of radioactivity in the thyroid gland than in normal persons.

Hyperthyroidism is a very treatable disease. Forms of treatment include surgery for removal of part of the gland, radioactive iodine, and chemicals that block the formation of thyroid hormones.

In general, the pendulum has swung away from surgery with subtotal removal of the thyroid gland to the use of radioactive iodine. Often the person with advanced thyroid disease is treated by several means. Antithyroid drugs that block the formation of new hormone are used and chemicals given to modify the effects in the body of the excess thyroid hormone already manufactured. A single dose of radioactive iodine is then given which, usually over several weeks, has the desired effect on the thyroid gland. Additional doses may be required in some cases.

In young children, surgical removal of the gland is preferred to use of a radioactive substance, which although safe for an adult may expose the youngster to additional risks. In pregnancy, the antithyroid drugs, such as propylthiouracil, may be used so as not to subject the thyroid of the fetus to a potentially toxic dose of radioactivity.

Most often, an endocrinologist, a physician who is a specialist in treating diseases of the endocrine glands, assists in advising the best treatment for the particular patient. The risk of many years later developing an underactive thyroid with both radioactive iodine or surgery is significant. This can be easily monitored by periodic blood tests and corrected by administering thyroid hormone tablets when necessary.

Hypothyroidism. Hypothyroidism develops when the

thyroid gland fails to produce an adequate amount of thyroid hormone. The disease may develop as a consequence of pituitary disease, which causes a failure of thyroid stimulating hormone production. More commonly, hypothyroidism is simply a primary failure of the thyroid gland itself.

The disease has a wide range of symptoms, depending on whether it is detected early, when symptoms are minimal and not specific, or later, when the patient may go into coma. Many obese persons diagnose themselves as suffering from an "underactive thyroid gland," hoping their difficulty stems from a glandular problem, "sluggish thyroid," and not from their dietary escapades and overindulgences. Tiredness, weakness, lack of energy and pep, symptoms that do occur in hypothyroidism, are common in many diseases as well as in psychoneurotic states.

Hypothyroidism can be present at birth, producing the disease known as *cretinism*. In adults, a typical patient with hypothyroidism has a dull, expressionless face, with coarse features, including puffiness of the eyelids and face. The speech is slow and hoarse. The patient complains of weakness and lethargy, poor memory and difficulty in concentrating, intolerance to cold weather, weight gain and constipation, and possibly changes in the hair and skin, including hair loss and thickening and coarseness of the skin.

On examining the patient, the tongue is thickened and enlarged; the face and skin are pale; characteristic changes in the tendon reflexes are present.

Laboratory studies that confirm the diagnosis include a reduced blood thyroxin level and a slow radioactive thyroid uptake. In this case, the level of radioactivity concentrated by the thyroid gland in 24 hours is below normal. Other findings commonly seen in hypothyroidism include an elevated cholesterol level in the blood and the presence of a mild to moderate anemia.

Treatment of this disorder is always successful and simple. Patients can be returned to normal by replacement of thyroid hormone. Many types of thyroid medication are available and have included crude thyroid hormone extracted from animal thyroids, improved animal thyroid extracts, synthetic thyroxin or thyronine, and combinations of the latter two. An adult requires two to three grains of thyroid extract or its equivalent to maintain a normal, or *euthyroid* state. Medication is required for the duration of the patient's life once the diagnosis of hypothyroidism is established.

Thyroid Tumors.   Tumors or masses may be either benign or malignant (cancerous). Goiters, discussed above, are almost always benign. Although several different forms of malignancies can develop in the thyroid gland, most nodules will be benign growths called *adenomas*.

In general, the common malignant tumors of the thyroid grow slowly. Nodules which are quite firm, are enlarging rapidly, and have associated enlargement of lymph glands are more likely to be malignant. Scans of the thyroid gland are made with radioactive iodine to aid in evaluating solitary thyroid nodules. The iodine is injected and a picture of the thyroid gland and the nodule is made because the radioactive iodine concentrates in the thyroid gland. A *cold nodule,* one that fails to concentrate the radioactive iodine, is likely to be malignant, in contrast to a nodule that picks up the iodine. Useful information about the thyroid gland is also provided by the use of ultrasound.

Surgical excision of a solitary, suspicious nodule is the treatment of choice. More advanced disease may require more extensive surgery. Certain thyroid cancers spread to distant sites, including lung and bone. Some of these retain their ability to concentrate iodine and can be treated with higher, therapeutic doses of radioactive iodine, which will kill the cancerous cells. Only 0.4 percent of all cancer deaths are due to thyroid cancer.

Thyroiditis.   The thyroid can be involved in an inflammatory disorder called thyroiditis. The condition may follow a mild respiratory infection. Viruses are felt to be responsible for many cases but this is not proved. Most often no cause is found. Women are affected much more often than men.

In acute cases, the patient may complain of tenderness over the neck in the thyroid region, accompanied by chills, fever, and malaise. The patient may be relatively asymptomatic except for swelling of the gland. A chronic form, called *Hashimoto's* thyroiditis, develops more insidiously as an enlarging goiter with pressure symptoms in the neck.

Many persons with thyroiditis eventually develop hypothyroidism and require thyroid hormone.

Adrenal Glands

The two adrenal glands lie in the flank area, capping the

upper poles of both kidneys. The name itself means "adjacent to the kidneys." Anatomically, three separate regions can be distinguished in the gland, which weighs around 5 grams. Very important hormones, called *steroids*, are produced from cholesterol by the adrenal glands.

The corticosteroids, the most widely known of the steroids, perform many functions that are vital for normal health. In fact, all organs of the body in some way require their presence. The energy necessary for all body reactions is produced in the cells ultimately by the combustion of sugars. Since we normally eat only several times a day, during periods of fasting, protein stored in the liver is broken down and converted into useful energy forms under the influence of steroids. Steroids are important in fat metabolism, muscle performance, moderating inflammatory reactions and antibody production, and the response of connective tissue to injury and repair.

The synthesis of many steroid derivatives has brought them into widespread use in clinical medicine, and steroids are sometimes heralded as miracle drugs. Probably every disease process of known or unknown origin has been treated by steroids of this class. Despite their overuse, there are many bonafide uses for corticosteroids.

Steroids have proved quite helpful in treating contact dermatitis, including poison ivy, psoriasis, neurodermatitis, and many nonspecific skin rashes. Other areas of proved value include asthma, certain blood diseases, kidney, gastrointestinal, brain, and blood vessel disorders, which have in common inflammation, and at times, production of abnormal proteins called immune complexes, which can damage tissues, especially small blood vessels.

Mineralocorticoids control the process of sodium (salt) reabsorption or loss in the kidneys as well as that of potassium.

Androgens and estrogens, the respective sex hormones of men and women, although produced chiefly by the testes and ovaries, are also made in the adrenal glands. Approximately two-thirds of androgens are formed by the testes (testosterone is the main product), and the rest are made in the adrenal gland and are known as weak androgens, in contrast to testosterone. In one sense, sex is an artificial separation if one uses hormone production, for every male manufactures some female hormone, and every female produces some weak male hormones.

The growth of facial hair, a source of embarrassment and

frustration to women, occurs in most women to some extent; but women with dark complexions may have more noticeable facial hair, or *hirsutism*. This problem may be due to the presence of increased amounts of the normally present adrenal androgens in some women.

Androgens account for the larger muscle mass, body and facial hair, and sperm maturation in males. Estrogens induce the characteristic body shape of females, including breast development, and together with progesterone, control the various events of the female menstrual cycle.

Disorders of the adrenal gland are quite uncommon. Just as in the case of the thyroid gland, adrenal problems can be due to excess production of steroid hormones, called hyperadrenalism or *Cushing's disease*, or underproduction of steroid hormones, hypoadrenalism or *Addison's disease*.

Hyperadrenalism (Cushing's Disease). Harvey Cushing (1869-1939), the great American neurosurgeon, described a disease due to excess production of steroid hormones by the adrenal gland. He believed the disturbance was caused by a pituitary tumor producing an excess of ACTH (adrenocorticotropic hormone), the pituitary hormone that stimulates the activity of the adrenal gland. Most cases of Cushing's syndrome are due to excess growth—an increase in size called hyperplasia—of both adrenal glands. Approximately a third of cases occur because of tumors of the adrenal gland, of which about half are malignant.

Symptoms of Cushing's disease are caused by the excess production of the various steroids (cortisol), androgens, and mineralocorticoids. Associated with excess cortisol is a particular type of obesity that involves the trunk but spares the extremities. Fat deposition in the nape of the neck leads to the so-called buffalo-hump. The face is round or moon-shaped. There are striae or purplish stretch marks over the abdomen and extremities. The skin is thin and the complexion ruddy. There is marked muscle wasting and weakness. Excess cortisol also produces bruising and leads to diabetes mellitus and hypertension. Bone thinning or osteoporosis occurs, and fractures of the spine may develop.

Androgen excess leads to the development of acne, increased body and facial hair, baldness, and deepening of the voice.

Electrolyte (salt) disturbances, that is, reduced potassium and retention of sodium, associated with hypertension, occur because of mineralocorticoid excess.

The diagnosis of hyperadrenalism requires laboratory documentation of excess steroid production in the urine and blood. Attempts to suppress steroid production by using various drugs often permits differentiation between hyperplasia and tumor.

Once a diagnosis is confirmed, surgical exploration and removal of both glands is curative in cases of hyperplasia. This procedure produces the disorder discussed below, hypoadrenalism, unless replacement treatment with the essential hormones is given. This consists of cortisone or similar drugs as well as a mineralocorticoid drug. Recently, a drug, cyproheptadine, has been used successfully in treating Cushing's disease.

Hypoadrenalism (Addison's Disease).   Hypoadrenalism can occur because of failure of the pituitary to produce adequate ACTH, so that the adrenal glands cannot manufacture steroid hormones. Addison's disease, named after the famous English physician (1793-1860) who described the disease, is a failure of the adrenal gland to produce its hormones despite a normal pituitary gland.

The disease may be difficult to diagnose depending on the degree of adrenal failure. Symptoms may develop only during a stressful event such as surgery, acute infection, or trauma when normally the body requires increased levels of steroids.

Addison described the disease as follows: "The leading and characteristic features of the morbid state to which I would direct attention are anemia, general languor and debility, remarkable feebleness of the heart's action, irritability of the stomach, and a peculiar change in the color of the skin."

Increased skin pigmentation all over the body, poor appetite, nausea and vomiting, weakness and dizziness, small heart-size, and a low blood pressure are features of hypoadrenalism.

If the diagnosis is suspected, measurement of the steroids in blood and urine samples will reveal the characteristic reduced levels. Failure of the steroid values to improve after ACTH hormone is given establishes the inability of the adrenal glands to function properly.

Treatment is by replacement therapy, which includes cortisone or its equivalent and a mineralocorticoid, 9-alpha fluorohydrocortisone (Fluorinef). With such a regimen, patients are usually able to lead normal lives.

Diabetes Mellitus

Four million Americans have diabetes mellitus, and half of them don't even suspect it. Of those who do know they have this disease, a large percentage are unaware of the importance of controlling it and of the proper treatment to prevent early death or disabling conditions. On the basis of numbers of people involved, potentially serious complications and practicality of medical management, diabetes mellitus rates with high blood pressure as one of the two most important health areas in which the public needs to be educated.

The name of the disease tells us something about its nature. "Diabetes" means fountain and "mellitus" sweet, a natural name for a condition often characterized by passing large amounts of urine which contains sugar. Diabetes mellitus is a disease primarily of carbohydrate metabolism; that is, the basic abnormality is in the way the diabetic's body handles sugar. This leads to other metabolic changes which cause complications in many parts of the body and can result in serious symptoms and even death. To understand the fundamentals of diabetes mellitus, we must first learn about carbohydrate metabolism.

About 50 percent of the carbohydrate in the average American's diet is present in the grains and vegetables we eat (starches), and another 25 percent is in our table sugar (both cane and beet); most of the rest is taken in as milk and milk products, fruits, honey, molasses, and maple and corn syrup. All these various carbohydrates are digested and absorbed into the blood as simple sugars, and finally converted, for all practical purposes, almost entirely into glucose.

Glucose is brought to the muscles and to the liver, where it is stored as glycogen. In the muscles it is used for the energy of muscle contraction and, therefore, work, while in the liver it is used to power the chemical work of the liver. Glucose is also converted into fat, and some enters into the metabolism of protein. The glucose in the liver is released back into the blood as needed in order to keep up a normal blood sugar level. This is necessary because glucose is continually entering all the cells of the body, where it is consumed as fuel for the chemical processes of life. As the glucose leaves the blood to enter cells, it must be replenished at the same rate.

Normally, the blood glucose level (in medical slang, the blood sugar) is between 60 and 100 milligrams per 100 milliliters of blood, but it may rise to 150 or 160 after a meal as the digested carbohydrates are absorbed into the blood. There are many avenues of control of the blood sugar, but the most important is through the hormone insulin, manufactured in certain cells of the pancreas. When the blood sugar begins to climb above ideal levels, these cells release insulin in amounts calculated to drop the blood sugar back to normal. On the other hand, when the blood sugar level begins to drop, insulin secretion is decreased or stopped, so that the blood sugar can climb back to normal as the liver releases glucose into the circulation. Actually, many other controls, especially including the hormones epinephrine and glucagon, are involved in this process, but here we are concerned with the effects of insulin.

The major defect in persons who have diabetes mellitus is a lack of proper insulin activity. We do not know the cause of diabetes mellitus, although there is a vast amount of information accumulated about the metabolic defects that go with this disease. In most cases, it is not due simply to failure of the specialized pancreatic cells to make insulin, but in all cases, the patient's body acts as though it had not enough insulin for his needs.

Diabetes mellitus may occur at any age, although it is more common in middle-aged and older persons. When it develops in children, the onset is usually sudden, most often with an infection, such as pneumonia, or with diabetic acidosis, which is discussed below. In adults the disease may be present for a long time without the person involved ever knowing he has it. It is often first suspected by finding glucose (sugar) in the urine or an elevated blood sugar level on a routine examination. Frequently a person with diabetes will first consult a doctor because of excessive thirst, increased amounts of urine, weight loss despite a good appetite, visual disturbances, or repeated infections. Another way in which the diagnosis is suspected is in the diagnostic work up of a person who has had a heart attack or a stroke.

Finding sugar in the urine does not automatically mean that diabetes is present. Some families have renal glycosuria, a condition in which their urine contains sugar even with the blood sugar within normal limits. An elevated fasting blood sugar level, that is, a blood sugar determination done when the patient has not had anything to eat overnight, usually means that diabetes is present, but even this is not definite, as some other conditions can raise the blood sugar level. Often a person with mild diabetes can have a normal fasting blood sugar level, but have an excessive elevation after taking food. Because of this, a better screening test for diabetes is the postprandial blood sugar, that is, a sample taken two hours after eating a meal containing large amounts of carbohydrates. This should be close to the fasting level in normal people, but persons with even mild diabetes may still have a significant elevation in the glucose level at this time.

A more sensitive means of making the diagnosis of diabetes mellitus is the glucose tolerance test. This measures how the person's body handles carbohydrates. A fasting blood sugar level is obtained, and then the patient is given a measured amount of carbohydrate depending on his body weight, usually glucose in a flavored solution. Blood is then tested one half hour, one hour, two hours, and three hours later. Normally, the blood sugar will not rise above 170 milligrams at any time and will be back to normal by two hours and a little under the fasting level at three hours because the elevated blood level will stimulate insulin secretion. If the blood sugar level is above 170 milligrams or is not back to normal by the end of two hours, then the person on whom the test is being done is said to have diabetes mellitus.

Treatment. The patient's cooperation is extremely important in the treatment of diabetes mellitus. It is essential that he or she understand as much as possible about this disease. The goals of treatment are to keep the blood sugar as normal as possible, to attain and maintain normal body weight, and to prevent complications. Complications are potentially fatal or disabling and will be discussed below.

Diet is by far the most important factor in treatment. Many persons with this disease are overweight, and it is imperative to bring them back to an ideal body weight. The initial dietary treatment has this as its goal. It is often discouraging at first, because it means existing on less than the usual amount of calories to carry out the day's work. However, once the normal weight is reached, the calories in the diet are adjusted so that the patient maintains his weight at that level. This is usually a satisfying amount of food and with knowledge and experience can be a delicious and varied diet. The amount of carbohydrate is controlled and may approximate that of the average American diet, which consists of 40 to 50 percent of carbohydrate.

Most doctors use the American Diabetic Association dietary

plan. This divides all available foods into six types and lists amounts that can be interchanged within each type. This is a very practical form of dietetic treatment and can be understood by all persons of average intelligence.

In many diabetics, especially older ones, the disease can be controlled by dietary measures alone. However, it is sometimes necessary to prescribe medications. Insulin will be necessary for almost all younger diabetics and for many older diabetics whose disease cannot be controlled by diet or other drugs. Since insulin is digested in the stomach, it cannot be taken in pill form. It must be injected under the skin. There are other medications which are not insulin, but which act to drop the blood sugar level. Although the tablets are certainly much more convenient, they are not the same as the naturally produced insulin, and it is possible that there may be a higher incidence of cardiovascular disease in persons who have used the oral hypoglycemic agents (anti-diabetic drugs) for long periods of time. Some doctors feel these drugs lull the patient into a false sense of security and cause them to neglect their diets. If their use is necessary, however, they are considered sufficiently safe.

Several kinds of insulin are available. Regular insulin acts rapidly and is used up fairly rapidly, so that although it is excellent for emergency treatment, it really isn't practical for everyday use, since it would involve several injections daily. Long-acting insulin of various sorts is available, usually with an action of approximately 24 hours, so that a single daily injection in the morning can suffice. Dosage must be worked out for each individual.

Persons taking insulin can drop their blood sugar levels too low if they do not take in the usual amount of carbohydrate for that day or if they burn up excessive amounts with more exercise than they are accustomed to. When the blood sugar level drops too low, it can cause hypoglycemic reactions or insulin reactions, which can be quite unpleasant and may even be dangerous. Mild reactions may consist only in some nervousness and sweating, but a more severe reaction can lead to unconsciousness. Sometimes a person may act as though he were drunk during an insulin reaction, and people have even been jailed during such a reaction. Diabetics who use insulin should carry some sugar with them so that they can take it to avert reactions before they become serious. For severe reactions, an injectable drug, called glucagon, provides a prompt antidote for an insulin reaction.

Complications.   Almost all of the organs of the body can be affected by long-standing or poorly controlled diabetes mellitus. Diabetes is not just a disease of blood sugar, and the metabolic abnormalities take their main toll on the blood vessels.

Patients with diabetes develop early atherosclerosis leading to an increased likelihood of other blood vessel diseases, including heart disease and myocardial infarction, cerebrovascular disease, such as stroke, and diseases of the blood vessels in the legs. Similar changes in the blood vessels of the kidneys cause altered kidney function, and scarring of the glomeruli, the basic filtering network of the kidneys, can cause kidney failure. Diabetes is a leading cause of blindness.

Other tissues commonly involved include the peripheral nerves and the autonomic nervous system. Damage to the peripheral nerves causes impaired sensation in the hands and feet. Dysfunction of the autonomic nervous system can cause diarrhea and impaired absorption of nutrients from the gastrointestinal tract.

A major problem in diabetes mellitus is the development of *diabetic acidosis*, a condition that is fatal unless vigorous measures are undertaken to reverse the metabolic abnormalities.

Diabetic acidosis usually develops either in persons whose diabetes is not controlled because the diet is neglected or he or she does not take the prescribed insulin, or in someone whose diabetes is usually controlled, but who develops a complicating illness such as a viral gastroenteritis or an upper respiratory infection. Insulin deficiency, either relative or real, causes the blood sugar levels to rise, and inadequate glucose utilization leads the body to use fatty acids from its own fat stores as an alternative source of energy. Fatty acids are broken down to various acid substances by the liver (ketone bodies) and accumulate excessively in the blood, and this is called acidosis. The rising glucose levels in the blood cause increasing excretion by the kidneys with resulting losses of glucose, salts, and water, so that the person becomes dehydrated and eventually lapses into coma.

Usually, the patient is seen in an emergency room at the hospital, where the diagnosis is established. Besides a high blood sugar level, the doctor will find ketone bodies in the blood, and abnormal body electrolytes, including a reduced bicarbonate level, a low sodium level and an increase in the serum potassium.

Over the first few hours, several liters of dilute salt solutions are given intravenously to correct the dehydration and improve the circulation. Simultaneously, injections of regular insulin are given intravenously at frequent intervals to lower the blood sugar and to correct the acidosis. Frequent measures of the electrolytes, blood sugar, and acid level or pH of the blood are carried out, and additional amounts of insulin are given as well as various fluid mixtures to correct any deficits. After several hours and usually within 24 hours most of the abnormalities have been partially to fully corrected, and the development of hypoglycemia or a low blood sugar level has to be prevented by adding sugar to the intravenous fluids. Once the patient has stabilized and is out of danger, any precipitating factor, such as an infection, is treated.

Edema

Edema is a term used to describe the accumulation of fluid in the tissues of the body. It is usually detected by firmly pressing a thumb or fingertip on the skin, usually of the foot or leg, which leaves a visible indentation on the surface of the skin. Edema generally occurs in the dependent portions of the body because of the effect of gravity. In an ambulatory person, edema forms in the ankles or lower legs, and a bedridden patient may have edema of the tissues of the back. Edema may occur around the eyes or periorbital tissue because of the looseness of the skin in this area.

The causes of edema are numerous. Patients with a low level of plasma proteins develop edema because these proteins, particularly albumin, serve to keep fluid in our blood vessels and out of body tissues. Patients who have certain types of kidney diseases lose large amounts of protein in their urine and may develop edema not only of the ankles and legs, but of much of the body. Persons with severe liver disease develop edema and abdominal swelling with fluid, called ascites, for several reasons, including an inability to manufacture plasma proteins. Congestive heart failure is often first diagnosed in a patient with ankle swelling or edema which occurs because the weakened heart muscle is unable to pump blood adequately. The above conditions generally are associated with other symptoms. Medical attention is required to diagnose the underlying illnesses so that the appropriate treatment can be given.

The most common form of edema occurs in females. It tends to be worse around the menstrual period, and some women gain several pounds because of fluid accumulation. In these cases, the cause is probably some hormonal influence on salt and water retention. Edema generally is not present in the morning but develops during the day. It may also occur in persons who do a lot of standing, especially if they are immobile for much of the time. Edema is primarily due to retention of salt, which leads to water retention. Thus edema formation may be largely prevented in some persons if they avoid a large salt intake and salt-containing foods such as pork products, cold cuts, peanuts, and potato chips.

If edema does not respond to salt restriction and is troublesome, for example, if shoes do not fit and the body feels too bloated or full, diuretics or fluid pills can be given. These act by increasing the kidney's excretion of salt and water. Many women need to take diuretics only around their menstrual period. Others require them on a regular basis, but generally, a pill every second or third day will control edema formation and the side effects of the drug will be minimal. Excessive use of diuretics tends to cause increased loss of potassium from the tissues. This may cause weakness as well as disabling muscle cramps. Patients who are taking certain types of heart medications such as digitalis may develop serious complications if diuretics are used excessively or if proper potassium balance is not maintained with supplemental potassium medications.

Symptoms you should know about:

Endocrine disease may cause all sorts of symptoms, few of which indicate a specific hormonal disorder. The thirst, urinary frequency, urination during the night, and weight loss of diabetes are the commonest endocrine symptoms. Weakness, easy fatigability, menstrual irregularities, obesity (rarely), sexual dysfunction, and increased body hair are complaints that often start a search for a disease of the endocrine system in adults.

GYNECOLOGY 7

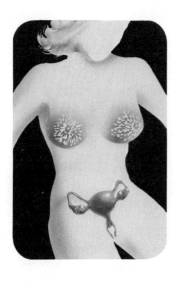

The Menstrual Cycle

Much folklore exists in various cultures regarding the significance of menstruation. Many women are misinformed concerning some aspect of the monthly period or *menses*.

Most women experience periods or menstruation at regular intervals during their approximately 30 reproductive or childbearing years. Periods represent the complex interplay of various hormones produced by the pituitary gland and ovaries on the uterus or womb. The object of these hormonal actions is to produce an egg from the ovary which, if fertilized by a sperm, can be satisfactorily imbedded and nourished in the lining of the uterus to form a healthy fetus. When no conception occurs, the hormonal balance achieved during this cycle wanes, and the inner lining of the uterus, called the *endometrium*, is shed, producing several days of bloody flow or discharge called a period.

Periods usually begin around age 12 to 14 years, although in certain races they can start as early as 9 years. It is not unusual for periods to start as late as 17 years of age. The exact event that triggers the onset of sexual maturation and periods is unknown. The hypothalamus, an area of the brain located near the pituitary gland, somehow, perhaps chemically, instructs the pituitary gland to make hormones that affect the female reproductive organs, the ovaries. (See illustration 9.) *Follicles* are located in the ovaries and begin to develop and mature under the influence of a pituitary hormone called FSH (follicle stimulating hormone). The maturing follicle in turn produces the female hormone called *estrogen*. Estrogen production leads to breast development, but here the hormone is important for its effect on the endometrium or inner lining of the uterus. Another pituitary hormone called LH (luteinizing hormone) together with FSH stimulates ovulation, when one follicle ruptures and discharges its egg, or *ovum*. Generally, only one follicle matures and ovulates during a cycle; the others degenerate. Ovulation usually occurs midway through the menstrual cycle, approximately two weeks before the period begins. The egg then travels through the *fallopian tubes* toward the uterus. Successful fertilization or impregnation of the egg by sperm usually occurs during the passage through the fallopian tube to the uterus. Meanwhile the ruptured follicle cyst, now called a *corpus luteum*, manufactures another hormone called *progesterone*, which further affects the glandular structure of the lining of the uterus or endometrium. If after four to six days, fertilization of the egg has not occurred, the activity of the corpus luteum regresses, the levels of both estrogen and progesterone drop, new follicles begin to develop in the ovaries under the influence of FSH, and the period begins. During each cycle, the endometrium is prepared to receive a fertilized egg; if this does not occur, the endometrium is shed, and another cycle is begun.

The menstrual cycle culminating in the period may be quite regular, occurring at 26- to 30-day intervals in some women. Others have a wide variation in their cycles, with periods occurring at 3- to 6-week intervals, or they may even miss periods for a month or two or longer. The period itself can be as short as one or two days or as long as seven or eight days. Some women report scant flow all during a period, and some have a heavy flow, usually for the first or second day of the period. Periods can be quite painful, especially for the first or second day, or only a minor discomfort. Any of these normal variations from woman to woman can cause concern. Painful periods (dysmenorrhea), irregular periods, heavy flow during periods (menorrhagia), scanty flow during periods, or absence of periods (amenorrhea) are problems often brought to the physician.

Irregular Periods.   There is nothing magical about a 28-day menstrual cycle, although the association with the lunar calendar is noted in some cultures. Certain women are quite "regular" and enjoy predictable periods. Others have menstrual cycles that occur sporadically and even stop for many months without the woman being pregnant or menopausal. It is quite common for a young woman to develop irregular periods during times of stress and major changes in her lifestyle. This typically occurs when a student leaves home to attend college or it may be associated with marked weight loss during dieting. Most women fall into an intermediate position, with periods occurring fairly regularly until approaching the menopause, when they become more and more irregular.

Regular periods are important to women who practice a form of birth control called *rhythm.* The rhythm method attempts to prevent conception by abstinence from sexual relations during the optimal time for pregnancy to occur—

Female Reproductive System:
Side View (sagittal section) of
genital organs and relationship to
the urinary bladder, urethra, and rectum

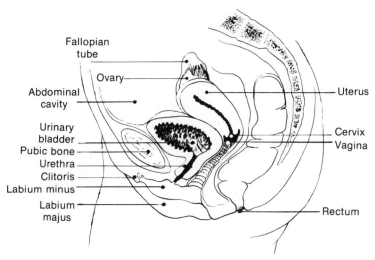

Illustration 9

several days before ovulation and several days following ovulation. This form of birth control, abstinence during the time the egg can be fertilized, can be practiced with some success only when a woman's menstrual cycle is regular.

Absence of Periods.   Amenorrhea or the absence of periods can be a primary problem, meaning periods have never occurred, or secondary, meaning periods have stopped after a series of them. Primary amenorrhea is a relatively rare disorder and requires a detailed evaluation of the normal functioning of the pituitary gland, ovaries, and the female organs, including the uterus. Secondary amenorrhea is relatively common, and as indicated above, can be a temporary event associated with a major stressful experience. Whenever a physician is asked to evaluate the cessation of periods in a sexually active woman of reproducing age, his first consideration is pregnancy—the most common cause of skipped period(s). This diagnosis can be substantiated by a pelvic examination which allows evaluation of the size of the uterus, which enlarges during pregnancy. A positive pregnancy test from a urine specimen allows corroboration of the physical findings of pregnancy. Early in pregnancy the urine test can still be negative, but this test often is positive when the diagnosis cannot be made from the size of the uterus on pelvic examination.

Periods also stop, although usually not abruptly, when the menopause is reached and the ovaries no longer ovulate and support the uterine changes described previously. A woman's age at menopause varies considerably. Usually she is in her mid- to late forties, but it may occur in the thirties to the mid-fifties.

Painful Periods.   Most women experience some degree of discomfort slightly before or during the period. Weight gain because of the retention of fluids is caused by the hormones involved, and lower abdominal cramps or pressure with low backache is quite common.

A condition called *endometriosis,* in which endometrial tissue is outside of the usual location in the uterus and responds to the cyclical character of the period, is associated with painful periods.

Most women readily admit to being more irritable and grouchy during their periods. Some do experience considerable discomfort, to the point where pain medications are necessary; they may have to lie down for part of the day to get relief from the pain and cramps. A heating pad applied to the lower abdomen often decreases the distress. Particularly painful periods account for considerable absenteeism from work, especially during the first or second day of the menses. Women with emotional problems are prone to report a greater degree of disability and distress as well as accentuation of their emotional problems during their periods. Undoubtedly, many women with greater stoicism tend to play down any distress associated with their period and carry on their normal activities unimpeded by pain.

Infertility

Infertility is the inability to achieve pregnancy after regular sexual relations for a period of at least one year. *Sterility*, the inability to conceive, is the term applied when an individual has some factor preventing conception (a woman who has had a hysterectomy—removal of her uterus—or a man who has had a vasectomy).

It is estimated that between 10 and 15 percent of all married couples in this country have a problem with infertility. Some have no demonstrable cause for their problem, and many women eventually conceive. In cases where a cause for infertility is found, approximately half are due to disturbances in the female partner and half to abnormalities in the male.

For most married couples wanting children, each barren and unfruitful month adds to the disappointment and frustration of their marriage. To the physician who works with an infertile couple, helping to solve their dilemma and enabling those with a correctable problem to conceive, is a most rewarding effort.

Attempts to unravel the numerous possible causes of infertility require the interest and cooperation of both partners. Both require medical examinations to rule out medical problems, such as thyroid disease. Most couples are encouraged to continue regular sexual relations, since their method of intercourse is seldom the cause of infertility.

The male patient undergoes an analysis of his *semen* (the liquid ejaculation from sexual relations) collected after several days of refraining from sexual relations. Sperm counts below 20 million are associated with sterility; counts between 20 million and 60 million can cause infertility.

The female undergoes a physical examination and a careful history including her menstrual history. If her husband has had a normal sperm analysis and no abnormalities are detected on the physical and pelvic examinations of the woman, further tests are done to determine whether ovulation takes place. Ovulation does not occur in every menstrual cycle. Several means of assessing ovulation are available. Normally, a slight temperature elevation occurs at the time of ovulation. This can be noted by recording the daily temperature first thing in the morning on a chart. The cervical mucus from the uterus shows a characteristic fern-like appearance under the microscope when ovulation takes place. The most sensitive way to determine whether ovulation takes place is to have a D & C (dilatation and curettage) or uterine scraping done right before an expected period. Analysis of the tissue obtained shows characteristic effects of progesterone produced by the corpus luteum of ovulation if it has occurred.

If evidence for ovulation is obtained, the next area of evaluation is the *fallopian tubes,* or uterine tubes which transport the egg to the uterus for implantation if the egg has been fertilized. If the tubes are damaged or scarred from previous infection, passage of the egg may be prevented and no pregnancy can occur. Evaluation of the tubes by various techniques, including passage of air or by injection of dye during x-ray exam, helps determine their patency. Blocked fallopian tubes usually develop from chronic pelvic infection caused by previous infections from gonorrhea, streptococci, or, less commonly, tuberculosis. The recent birth of a "test tube baby" carried out by a British team of doctors offers great promise for infertility caused by damaged fallopian tubes. An egg is removed surgically from the woman's ovary, fertilized by sperm, nourished in appropriate fluids, and implanted directly into the uterus.

Direct visualization of the ovaries by introducing a small instrument into the abdomen allows inspection of these glands. Sometimes, a surgical exploration and examination is done, especially when ovulation has not occurred. A specific condition exists where infertility is present and is associated with cystic ovaries, obesity, and increased body hair. Treatment at the time of surgery by partial resection of the ovaries usually leads to subsequent pregnancies.

If all studies are negative, and all systems appear to be functioning normally in both the husband and the wife, they are encouraged to continue their efforts to conceive. Sexual relations are especially likely to be successful at the time of ovulation. The woman is encouraged to keep a temperature chart and the husband to abstain from sexual relations for several days to have a maximal sperm level.

If significant reasons exist for infertility or sterility, the unlikelihood of conception is discussed with the couple. The majority of couples who desire children will accept the suggestion of adoption, contact an appropriate adoption agency, and patiently wait for a placement to be made.

If the husband is infertile or sterile, pregnancy can be induced by artificial insemination, using donor sperm that can be introduced by the physician.

The donor of the sperm should be in good physical health, emotionally stable, free of hereditary diseases, and intelligent.

Birth Control Measures

Birth control efforts have been practiced for thousands of years by mankind with various degrees of success. In ancient Egypt, the gum of the acacia plant, which contains lactic acid—a common ingredient of many current spermicides, was used to prevent pregnancy. Today, family planning is a major goal of many underdeveloped nations with too many mouths to feed. It is also widely accepted among many young couples in Western countries. For the latter, birth control is essential to limit the size of their families in order to provide maximal education and economic security for their children. In addition, sometimes there are philosophical considerations which include a family's responsibility to its total environment. The question of birth control is steeped with many religious, moral, and ethical considerations.

The most reliable method for birth control is refraining from sexual relations or abstinence. This practice obviously will have few adherents and warrants no further attention. However, the rhythm technique, mentioned in the section on the menstrual cycle and irregular periods is really a form of abstinence during the time of the menstrual cycle when ovulation and fertilization are most likely to occur. Since ovulation occurs on the average of the 14th day of the ideal 28-day cycle, but may occur from the 8th to the 18th day, practicing rhythm requires a well disciplined couple. Success with this technique varies considerably.

Another technique, premature withdrawal by the male before his ejaculation, also is successful, but requires interruption of intercourse and loss of part of the pleasurable sensation associated with sexual relations.

Mechanical Devices. Mechanical devices were much used, and quite successfully, prior to the advent of birth control pills.

Condoms, or rubberlike sheaths that are applied to the penis, prevent entry of sperm into the vagina. This technique, with nontearing and nonleaking condoms, works well but does involve lessening of the sexual pleasure to both partners.

The use of *diaphragms,* thin elastic discs, inserted into the vagina by the female, when used with various contraceptive jellies or foam which contain chemicals to interfere with sperm, is another highly safe technique. This requires a properly fitted and applied diaphragm.

Coils of various plastic and metal design can be inserted into the uterus by a physician and prevent pregnancy by interfering with implantation of a fertilized egg. In some women, especially those who have had frequent pregnancies, the risk of the coil falling out is real. An additional risk is perforation of the uterus by the coil which leads to serious abdominal infection and which requires surgical intervention to remove it. Coils are highly effective and have been used successfully by hundreds of thousands of women. Because they are a foreign body in the uterus, they may be associated with a lot of vaginal discharge, which can be a nuisance to some women.

Birth Control Pills. Birth control pills contain hormones that simulate a condition of pregnancy in the user and prevent ovulation or egg formation. The pills contain small amounts of the two hormones of the menstrual cycle, estrogen and progesterone. Two types are available, *combination* or *sequential* types. Combination birth control pills contain the two hormones together taken for 21 days. Sequential birth control pills contain two types of pills. The first type taken for most of the cycle contains estrogen only. For the last several days, progesterone is added to the second type of pill. This routine attempts to reproduce the way the body normally makes female hormones.

Birth control pills are generally taken for 21 days, then stopped, and the period takes place. The pills are resumed on the fifth day following the onset of the period. Birth control pills are virtually 100 percent effective if taken regularly.

Many women have reservations about their use. Some of these stem from guilt feelings in using birth control pills against accepted religious doctrines. Others are rightly concerned about dangerous short- and long-term side effects.

Birth control pills have undergone changes since their first introduction. The dose of estrogen has been reduced. Despite this, many women experience nausea and morning sickness on initiating their use. This generally decreases with their continued use. Birth control pills work because they simulate pregnancy. Breast enlargement regularly occurs as well as weight gain, and fluid retention develops and occasionally skin changes are noted. Most women tolerate and adjust to these changes and feel the freedom from an undesired pregnancy outweighs these side effects. Women who have hypertension or a tendency to high blood pressure should not use birth control pills. If headaches develop or if the blood pressure increases, birth control pills should be stopped. Several other categories of women should also not use birth control pills. Women who have had breast cancer or have a strong family history of breast cancer should not use these drugs even though there is no definite evidence to show birth control pills adversely affect the breasts or cause breast cancer. Women who have had phlebitis should not use the pills. Birth control pills do cause changes in the clotting of blood, as does pregnancy itself. There is a definite statistical risk of developing blood clots or phlebitis and the possibility of a pulmonary embolus. Yet, the overall safety of birth control pills exceeds the risks a woman faces during actual pregnancy. A question as to the association of birth control pills and strokes in young women has been raised. Women over the age of 40, especially if they have other risk factors for coronary artery disease, should avoid the pill.

In general, birth control pills provide a safe, secure means of birth control. It is recommended that women go off them for one or two months every couple of years so that periods will occur when the pills are finally discontinued. Birth control pills or anovulatory agents are also used for other female problems including correcting irregular menstrual cycles and treating endometriosis.

Another potential means of birth control is the so-called "morning after" pill. This involves using high doses of estrogen tablets for several days following intercourse and is reported to be successful. This form of birth control may be useful for the woman who engages in only sporadic sexual relations.

Tubal Ligation. Tubal ligation, or tying and removing part of the uterine tubes, is a surgical procedure performed in a hospital, which is effective as a permanent method for contraception and sterility. Tying off the tubes prevents the egg from reaching the uterus. The methods previously discussed prevent conception when used, but then allow for a planned pregnancy when discontinued. With a tubal ligation, future pregnancies are usually impossible. At times, women who require a Cesarean section and who are a poor risk for future pregnancy because of medical problems such as heart disease, undergo a tubal ligation as part of the operation.

Vasectomy. A very popular method of effective birth control is a *vasectomy.* This can be done as an out-patient procedure and involves ligating and removing part of the *vas deferens* through which sperm must travel to reach the penis during an ejaculation; the ejaculation still occurs after a vasectomy, but the secretion contains no sperm when the operation is properly performed.

For the couple certain of their family size, having fully considered the impact of an untimely death of a child, a vasectomy may be a good alternative to other forms of birth control. In a family with many children, and a mother with many childbearing years still ahead, this method may be the best one, if for various reasons she does not tolerate birth control pills.

The possibility of reuniting the severed ends of the vas is sometimes held out as a means of restoring fertility to the male. This has become a reality in up to 90 percent of cases by means of reconstructive microsurgery, which permits successful reuniting of the severed ends of the vas deferens.

Vaginal Discharge

The cervix is the neck of the uterus (womb), located in the deepest part of the vagina. There is an opening on its surface, called the os, through which menstrual flow passes. The tube-like passage through the cervix is called the cervical canal. Illustration 10 is a front view of a section cut through the uterus; compare it with the side view in illustration 9. Tiny glands in the cervix secrete mucus, which serves to plug the cervical canal and seal off the uterus to contamination from the vagina. Mucus secretion accompanies sexual stimulation and is necessary for the lubrication of the vagina during intercourse.

Uterus and Vagina

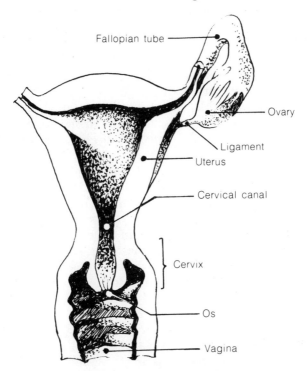

Fallopian tube

Ovary

Ligament

Uterus

Cervical canal

Cervix

Os

Vagina

Illustration 10

The amount of mucus produced by these glands varies considerably from woman to woman, and from time to time in the same person. It may be great enough to cause its discharge from the vagina. Normal mucus is clear or white, and its consistency varies from watery to jelly-like. In some women, nervous tension seems to increase the volume of mucus production.

When this normal discharge is annoying, as it sometimes can be, it can be controlled with douching. Plain water may be effective; a commercial preparation available at all drugstores, or a mild acid douche may also be used. An acid douche is made up of one tablespoonful of clear ("white") vinegar to one quart of water. A douche bag can be purchased at the drugstore, and is quite simple for almost all adult women to use.

We are often asked, "How often should I douche?" Unless specifically prescribed by a doctor for certain conditions, there is no universal answer to this question. Many women go through their lifetime without ever having used a douche, and depend on their usual bath for cleanliness. It is really a matter of taste and comfort. The vinegar douche can be overdone; daily use for long periods of time may be irritating. Most physicians feel there is no medical value to vaginal sprays, and their use may cause side effects.

Inflammation of the vagina causes vaginal discharge. Specific infections of the vagina result in the production of pus, and therefore varying degrees of discharge, burning, and itching. This may be due to the gonococcus (and the disease called gonorrhea); a bacterium called Hemophilus vaginalis; a yeastlike organism called Candida albicans (or Monilia); and a protozoan called Trichomonas vaginalis. The signs and symptoms of each of these infections may be different, and typically each causes a different appearance in the discharge. However, there are many individual variations, and an exact diagnosis can only be made by obtaining a fresh sample of discharge for examination and culture. This is extremely important, since treatment is different for each of these specific sorts of vaginitis.

Penicillin or a related antibiotic is necessary for gonorrhea. Flagyl tablets by mouth or special mercurial or iodine preparations applied to the vagina are the treatments for Trichomoniasis. Several sorts of vaginal tablets and creams are effective against Candidiasis. Sulfa or an antibiotic preparation in the form of vaginal tablets or cream is the treatment for Hemophilus vaginitis.

Recurrent cases of vaginitis or cases apparently resistant to treatment usually indicate that the cervix is involved. Minor surgical procedures are occasionally needed to correct this condition. The use of birth control pills may predispose a woman to vaginitis and make treatment difficult. Sometimes no specific cause can be found; this is called "non-specific vaginitis."

In post-menopausal women the absence of estrogen, the female hormone, may cause atrophy of the lining of the vagina. The wall becomes thinner and dry. This makes it inflamed and makes it susceptible to trauma during intercourse, which may become painful. It may also predispose to the infections mentioned above. Discharge or bleeding may occur. This condition, called atrophic vaginitis, requires the use of an estrogen cream in the vagina. The cream is preferable to estrogen by oral tablets, because small doses are effective, and the side effects of estrogens are minimized.

The Menopause
The menopause or cessation of periods occurs in middle-aged women. As discussed in the section on menstrual disorders, periods do not always end abruptly but may occur sporadically for a year or so before they end.

The menopause has two components: the physiological or body changes, and the psychological one—how a woman reacts to this event in the setting of other changes taking place in her life.

A definite change in the body accompanies the menopause. Normally, during the reproductive years, fluctuations in estrogen production by the ovaries cause changes in the secretion of the pituitary sex hormones. At the menopause, or even before the actual menopause, ovulation ceases in the ovaries and a gradual decline in estrogen production takes place. The drop in estrogen levels leads to an increased production of the pituitary sex hormones, giving rise to the characteristic symptoms of the menopause—hot flashes and sweats. The hot flashes usually involve the head, neck, and chest and are often followed by profuse sweating. The frequency and severity of these symptoms are quite variable, being negligible in some women, moderate in others, and quite severe in only a minority of women.

Despite the menopause, many women continue to produce estrogen hormone and do not require supplemental hormones. Over a period of years after the menopause, changes may occur in the skin, as well as in the genital area—vulva and vagina—due to decreased estrogen levels. The claims for the beneficial role of estrogen in preventing arteriosclerosis and decreasing vascular disease and in preventing degenerative arthritis are not based on solid evidence and are open to serious doubt.

For women who do experience frequent and severe hot flashes and sweats, replacement therapy with an estrogen preparation is useful. There is no advantage of monthly injection over tablets that contain estrogen hormone. Usually the tablets are given 3 weeks or 25 days out of the month to prevent constant stimulation of the breasts. If the menopausal symptoms are very disabling, hormones may have to be used daily. At times, vaginal bleeding follows withdrawal of the estrogen hormone. This is a matter of some concern, since it is also a symptom of serious uterine diseases.

Generally over a period of time, the dose of hormones may be reduced and then stopped. Contraindications to hormone treatment include previous breast or uterine cancer. Persons with hypertension who receive estrogen therapy require close supervision. There is recent evidence that estrogen treatment causes an increased incidence of uterine cancer when used in menopausal women.

Many symptoms that develop coincidentally with the menopause are not caused by any hormonal adjustments or deficiency states, but in fact represent various psychological and environmental factors.

To use the analogy of life as a book, the menopause represents the middle chapters of a woman's experience with much useful and fulfilling experiences ahead. Unfortunately, to some women, the menopause represents the end of the book. To these women, the cessation of childbearing potential brings with it a loss of self-esteem and worth, and marks the beginning of the end. Often, their role as mothers has also been undercut by the maturing of their children, who function quite independently. A marital relationship built entirely on their role as mothers may widen the gap in their marriages now that their children "no longer need them." These events together—lack of meaningful relationship with their husband, poorly developed image and capabilities outside their childbearing activities—brought closer to home by the onset of menopause, often produce a serious depression.

On the other hand, for many women, the end of childbearing and the growing up of their families provide new opportunities and a renewed sense of life. The ability to enjoy sexual relations free of responsibility of pregnancy allows for a continued active sex life. At the same time, less time is required at home for household chores; new vistas become possible as there is now the time to pursue personal goals, abandoned occupations, continued education, community activities, arts and crafts, and hobbies. A full and meaningful life lies ahead.

Postmenopausal Bleeding

Vaginal bleeding occurring in postmenopausal women requires investigation. As stated above, women on hormonal replacement treatment may experience bleeding when they are off the tablets for a few days. The bleeding may be due to uterine disease, which may be masked by attributing it to so-called withdrawal bleeding.

Cancer of the uterus cannot be detected consistently in the female by a cervical smear or Papanicolaou smear (Pap smear). In fact, the majority of Pap smears are negative or normal when uterine cancer is present. A Pap smear detects cancer only on the cervix or tip of the uterus where many cancers do develop. Vaginal bleeding in a postmenopausal woman therefore requires a careful pelvic examination which enables the physician to detect any enlargement of the uterus or ovaries as well as any abnormal mass. Dilatation and curettage (D & C), a scraping of the inside of the uterus, with examination of the removed tissue by a pathologist, allows determination of the cause of vaginal bleeding and the exclusion of cancer of the uterus.

Ovarian Cysts

The two ovaries often have small cysts when examined incidentally after a hysterectomy or during surgery for other reasons. In rare cases, ovarian cysts may produce abnormal amounts of hormones that cause generalized body changes. Most often, an enlarged mass or tumor is found in the area of the ovary as part of the pelvic examination during a routine physical examination. The mass may be quite large, and surgery is done to remove it. A certain percentage of ovarian masses or tumors are malignant, and prompt surgery and removal is the best means of achieving good results.

Dilatation and Curettage

Several times in the discussion of various gynecological problems, the performance of a D & C has been mentioned. This procedure is a scraping of the inner lining of the uterus and is performed with the patient under anesthesia, usually in the hospital. D & C's are performed for many different reasons, including the investigation of abnormal uterine bleeding (heavy periods, irregular periods, or postmenopausal bleeding). The tissue obtained from a scraping is helpful in the evaluation of an infertility problem, as previously discussed. Often, following the delivery of a child, abnormal bleeding persists, requiring a D & C. Removal of tissue that remains following a spontaneous abortion or miscarriage also requires a D & C.

The procedure is best performed by a gynecological surgeon, who first dilates the cervix to allow passage of a curette or scraper, which removes the tissue for evaluation by a pathologist.

Hysterectomy

A hysterectomy is an operation for removal of the uterus or womb. It is performed for various reasons. The most common one is excess vaginal bleeding and the finding of an enlarged uterus. Significant anemia may be caused by the heavy periods or frequent episodic bleeding. A cancer of the uterus has to be considered as a cause of vaginal bleeding especially in a postmenopausal woman, and can be revealed by a D & C.

Most often the enlargement is due to a *fibroid*, or benign growth of the muscle tissue of the uterus. Fibroids are often multiple and can grow to very large size. They are most often benign and will usually shrink after the menopause. If the bleeding is not too serious, fibroids may be observed at regular intervals to make sure their size is stable. A small number, less than one percent, become malignant and increase in size.

If bleeding in an enlarged uterus is persistent, and does not respond to a D & C, or efforts at hormonal manipulation, a hysterectomy is often done.

At the time of the hysterectomy, the surgeon may remove both ovaries and tubes, especially in a woman who is approaching the menopause or is postmenopausal. In a younger woman, part or an entire ovary may be left so that female hormones will continue to be produced, and to avoid a premature menopause. Often the appendix is removed at the time of surgery in an otherwise uncomplicated case.

The hysterectomy itself does not in any way prevent normal sexual relations following recovery from surgery. Subsequent pregnancies are of course impossible.

Symptoms you should know about:

Abnormal bleeding from the vagina may occur between monthly periods or may cause especially heavy but normally timed periods. Because of potentially serious causes, either sort of bleeding requires a medical opinion. Though most cases are not serious, the only way to be sure is to have a careful examination. Vaginal bleeding after the menopause should never be ignored.

DISEASES OF BONES AND JOINTS AND MUSCLE

8

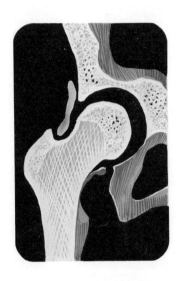

It is estimated that more than 16 million Americans have some form of rheumatic disease. Arthritis is the most serious of the rheumatic diseases, and there are many different kinds of arthritis. By far the commonest kind is *osteoarthritis*, or degenerative joint disease, followed by *rheumatoid arthritis*, which is potentially the most crippling kind, and then *gout*. We will discuss these three diseases in some detail later in this chapter as well as some conditions that are categorized as rheumatic diseases although they are not a form of arthritis, including the conditions that cause backache, the painful shoulder and bursitis.

The bones of our skeleton are joined to one another in various ways. The areas where the bones meet are called *joints*. For example, the knee joint is where the "thigh bone's connected to the leg bone," as the old song goes. Some joints are immobile (as where the various bones of the skull meet); some joints furnish a slight degree of motion (as discs between two vertebrae in the spine), but most joints are freely movable (as are the joints of our arms and legs). It is not surprising that many things can happen to these parts of our body, which do so much work, support our weight, are so often in motion, and are so exposed to injury. (See illustration 11.)

The Skeletal System

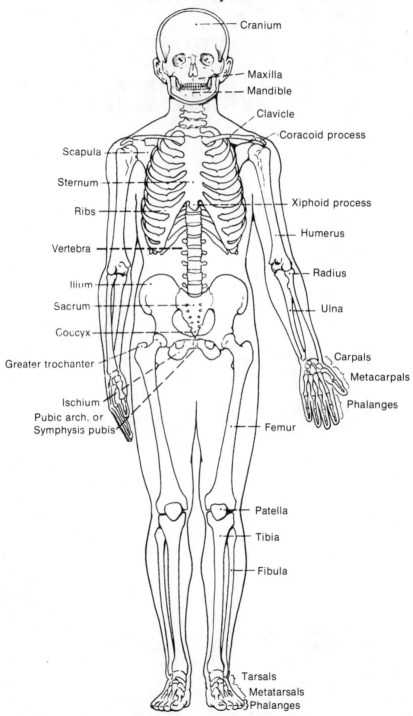

Illustration 11

Many diseases affect the joints. All sorts of infections can involve the joints, and when we think about it, it's a wonder that joint infections are so rare. Some intestinal diseases, like ulcerative colitis and regional enteritis, cause inflammation of the joints, as do many systemic diseases such as sarcoid, some blood conditions, endocrine (hormone) upsets, psoriasis, vitamin C deficiency, allergy, and a host of others.

Whatever the cause, the word *arthritis* means an inflammation of one or more joints. Other skeletal diseases may involve the bones, the muscles, and other tissue around the joints, but unless the joint itself is involved they can't be called arthritis. Arthritis and other diseases of the skeletal system are included in the family name of *rheumatic diseases*, and in common use the unscientific name *rheumatism* is used to refer to any of these painful afflictions of our bones and muscles, etc. *Rheumatic fever* is the name of a specific disease found most usually in children and young adults that involves the joints and other parts of the body, especially the heart, following an infection with a certain group of streptococcus germs. Rheumatologists, doctors who specialize in rheumatic diseases, recognize over 100 conditions that fall within their field.

Osteoarthritis or Degenerative Arthritis
The moving parts of our body are like those of any precision tooled machine. In time, continued use causes "wear and tear" or degenerative changes. Our bones and the joints, the hinges between bones, incur these changes of degeneration from the tremendous use that they undergo during our lifetime. Generally, persons involved in lots of hard physical work tend to develop more of this type of arthritis than those who are engaged in sedentary activities. Despite the best of care, our parts, or bones, inevitably show degenerative changes.

Degenerative bone disease is commonly seen in the hands and especially in women, who develop knobby projections off the sides of their distal interphalangeal joints adjacent to the fingertips. Despite this rather prominent appearance, most women are relatively asymptomatic and have full use of their hands. Often the tendency is inherited and a history of similar changes in other members of the family is obtained. Degenerative changes occur not only in the hands but in the neck, shoulders, back, hips, and knees.

The common types of degeneration occur at the articulations of joints where adjacent surfaces come into contact with one another. Irregular bony surfaces and projections develop. In the spine, degenerative changes produce a loss in height of vertebral bones. The bones, which normally are rectangular in shape on x-ray film, become concave and may become compressed or wedge shaped. These changes account for the increased round shoulders of the elderly and the loss of height, often several inches, that accompanies aging. In addition to loss of volume of bone, degenerative changes occur in the composition and thickness of bone. The surfaces of bones are no longer glistening and smooth but become roughened, and bone density decreases.

Many persons have little or no complaints, despite having advanced degenerative changes in bone, which would show up on x-rays. Others may have aching of shoulders, neck, hands, knees, hips, or back. The majority of persons with this type of discomfort achieve control of their symptoms with aspirin in its various forms. Cure of these changes is impossible, but control of discomfort usually is possible.

Rheumatoid Arthritis

A health survey by the United States government in the early 1960s found typical rheumatoid arthritis in one out of every 100 people examined and probable rheumatoid arthritis in another 2 out of 100. That means that perhaps 5 million Americans have some degree of rheumatoid arthritis. Most cases are chronic and not disabling, but these figures still represent a tremendous amount of suffering and time lost from work.

Rheumatoid arthritis is basically a disease of the "connective tissue" of the body, that is, those tissues that provide the supporting framework of the body and its internal organs. The three types of connective tissue are bone, cartilage, and fibroelastic connective tissue. Cartilage is a hard tissue (gristle to butchers and cooks) that forms the linings of joints, the front ends of our ribs, and the rings that keep open the upper air passages to the lungs. The fibroelastic connective tissue may be organized into compact bundles making up tendons and ligaments, or it may consist of sheets and collections of dense tissue which perform several functions. This tissue, for example, covers over the meaty organs (such as the capsule on the surface of the liver or spleen), makes up the great bulk of the walls of blood vessels, lies under the skin to give it strength and elasticity, and performs similar scaffolding jobs throughout the body.

The connective tissue in and around joints is mainly involved in rheumatoid arthritis, but sometimes tissue in other areas is affected, causing "extra-articular" (outside the joints) manifestations. In rare cases, these include inflammations of the heart or its lining, the lungs and pleura, not uncommonly the eye, fairly often the peripheral nerves, the skin, and so forth. When blood vessels are inflamed (vasculitis), virtually any part of the body can be damaged. Anemia and fever are common, reflecting the widespread nature of this disease in the body.

The cause of rheumatoid arthritis is unknown. Many clinical features suggest that an infectious agent is a possible cause, but intensive search for a single germ has been in vain. Several times, researchers have thought they have found the micro-organism that causes this disease, but never have they been able to prove it. Currently, scientific investigators suspect a virus or a similar very small organism called Mycoplasma as a cause.

Current evidence points to a possible immune mechanism for rheumatoid arthritis. The immune system was previously discussed in the section on asthma and allergy, where it was shown that an antigen or substance recognized as foreign by the body's lymphocytes stimulates production of antibodies or immunoglobulins. In asthma, the antigen was usually inhaled and the binding of it by antibody in the lung caused a release of various chemical mediators producing the clinical features of asthma. In rheumatoid arthritis many patients have in their blood as well as in joint fluid an antibody called rheumatoid factor, which belongs to the IgM class of immunoglobulins. This antibody is directed against another immunoglobulin which belongs to the class IgG. It has been postulated that slight alteration of the IgG molecules causes lymphocytes lining the joint surfaces to produce rheumatoid factor, which in combining with the IgG protein causes a release of enzymes within the joint, which then produces the inflammatory reaction leading to the changes seen in rheumatoid arthritis.

Although the disease is probably an ancient one and was named as long ago as 1859, it wasn't until the early years of the twentieth century that it was clearly distinguished from the arthritis due to tuberculosis (which, although rare now, used to be quite common) and other causes. Rheumatoid arthritis can occur at any age and involve any joint. Between two and three women are affected for every man.

Symptoms. Sometimes rheumatoid arthritis starts suddenly with the rapid onset of pain and swelling in the joints. In children, there is often a preceding period of unexplained fever and malaise or just plain sick feeling.

Most cases of rheumatoid arthritis, however, begin insidiously, that is, so slowly that the patient doesn't realize that something is wrong until he hasn't been well for a while. He realizes that he has had aching and stiffness for some time. These symptoms are usually worse on arising in the morning and disappear once the patient limbers up.

Adults with rheumatoid arthritis will then usually notice pain and swelling of the hands and feet, especially the middle set of knuckles on each hand. The large joints tend to become involved, especially the wrists, elbows, and knees. Indeed any joint can be affected. Over a period of time, the disease is roughly symmetrical, with joints on the left and right sides being similarly inflamed.

Most cases will improve by themselves, and from 15 to 20 percent will disappear completely. Unfortunately, however, some cases will progress relentlessly, and many of those who do improve at first will have exacerbations or flare-ups later.

As the disease advances, the pain, swelling, or deformity of the joints limits the victims' activities, and even permanent deformities can be produced. Although the crippling of far-advanced rheumatoid arthritis can result in a pain-racked, bedridden, deformed, chronic invalid with several destroyed joints, a well-motivated patient and modern therapy can prevent this gloomy eventuality in the overwhelming majority of cases.

The diagnosis of rheumatoid arthritis is made by finding a certain number of criteria, plus the absence of certain other conditions that also involve the joints. In other words, the doctor must rule out some diseases which mimic rheumatoid arthritis in that they cause arthritis, but which are basically different with different treatment and a different outlook. The most important positive findings are related to the arthritis itself: typical would be the presence of several large joints symmetrically inflamed. Other important points are the x-ray changes that may be present, blood tests for the rheumatoid factor, and examination of fluid which can be removed from an acutely inflamed joint through a needle. In early or mild cases of rheumatoid arthritis, the x-rays may be perfectly normal and the rheumatoid factor may not be present in the blood when the test is done.

Treatment. When the diagnosis of rheumatoid arthritis is made, the patient should be told that he has an unpredictable, chronic disease for which a good deal can be done. He should be instructed that treatment is not dramatic and that careful attention to homely details can often be the difference between being normally active and being disabled. Most of all the doctor should be encouraging, for it is only too easy to become discouraged by the slow improvement or even the flare-ups and complications that seem to come from nowhere. This is the classic example of the disease that the patient must "learn to live with."

In mild and moderate cases, simple aspirin is the single most important treatment measure. Aspirin, or acetylsalicylic acid as it is technically known, has many effects. It is not used here primarily for its pain-killing effect, but rather for its anti-inflammatory effect. Therefore, it must be taken at regular intervals every day and not simply when the patient is uncomfortable or in pain. Ideally, the largest amount that is effective and can be tolerated without side-effects should be used, usually between 10 and 15 tablets daily. If ringing in the ears, dizziness, or upset stomach appear, then the dosage should be adjusted downward.

In addition to aspirin, joint rest is a mainstay of treatment. This can mean temporary bed rest, as in someone with an acute process involving many joints. Often it means bandaging or splints to provide periods of immobilization and proper positioning of one or two joints. Physiotherapy usually consists of the use of various forms of heat (packs, diathermy, paraffin) and exercises designed to promote joint mobility and increase the strength of the muscles that support and move the involved joints.

Sometimes drugs other than aspirin are desirable. Chloroquine may be helpful, but it doesn't work quickly, and too much of this medication can affect the vision. This side-effect is usually only temporary but if ignored can in time result in irreversible loss of sight. Another drug that is sometimes helpful in producing a remission of rheumatoid arthritis is gold, which can be given in small amounts by injection over a long period of time. Other anti-inflammatory drugs are indomethacin (Indocin) and phenylbutazone (Butazolidin). Although stronger than aspirin, they are more likely to cause side-effects if used for long periods of time. Ibuprofen (Motrin) is a mild anti-inflammatory agent.

More severe cases may require the use of cortisone-type drugs, such as prednisone. These are often spectacularly successful. However, there are two drawbacks to what originally seemed to be a cure for rheumatoid arthritis. When the steroid (a name for the whole class of cortisone drugs) is stopped or the dose reduced, the disease may flare up, and the long-term use of large amounts results in serious side-effects. These side-effects include some life-threatening conditions, such as bleeding ulcers and diabetes; chronically disabling problems, such as thinness of bones with fractures; insomnia or psychosis; and obvious changes in the person's appearance, such as weight gain, "moonface," excess hair, and acne. If the dose can be kept low, then steroids can be used effectively for long periods.

Recently other medications helpful in treating rheumatoid arthritis have included alkylating agents, such as the very strong drugs used in treating several types of cancer, and immunosuppressive drugs. These must still be considered experimental, although in many cases they do show some promise.

Even when joints become permanently damaged by rheumatoid arthritis, operations may be available to correct or minimize the deformity and relieve inflammation and pain. Orthopedic surgery can now use artificial joints to replace diseased ones, such as the hip and knee.

It must be stressed that most cases of rheumatoid arthritis do not progress to this point and that patience and attention to detail make it possible for the patient to live quite fully with this disease. The natural course includes spontaneous improvement as well as flare-ups, and the overwhelming majority of cases are mild ones, which do not progress to cause serious problems.

Much has been written for the many sufferers from rheumatoid arthritis, most of which is nonsense and some of which is downright harmful. The fad diets that have been popular from time to time have made fortunes for their protagonists but have not helped the patients, who are always struggling for a sure cure.

Gout

Thanks to a comic strip called the "Katzenjammer Kids," most Americans over the age of 40 think that gout is a joke. The kids, Hans and Fritz, were irrepressibly mischievous and delighted in tormenting the patriarchal Captain, who was always portrayed with one foot swathed in bandages and elevated on a stool. The least movement would cause excruciating pain, and many cartoons were devoted to the Captain's roaring at the Kids' latest trick to get him to chase them. The young readers grew up thinking gout was a rare disease, caused by eating and drinking too much, that occurred in funny old men. About 275 out of every 100,000 Americans have found out that gout is no joke, and that they have it.

The name gout comes from the Latin word *gutta*, for drop, and is derived from the fact that in the thirteenth century, when the term was coined, it was thought that gout was due to a poison entering the inflamed joint drop by drop. Hundreds of years later it has been shown that this idea really reflects the facts and that acute gouty arthritis is caused by the precipitation of uric acid in the joints.

Most cases of gout begin suddenly in previously healthy persons, usually men, almost always over the age of 30. The victim initially feels a severe pain in the base of the big toe (the first metatarsal joint). Over the next few hours the area becomes swollen, hot, and reddened, and the pain gets even worse, aggravated by movement, touching the toe, or standing up on that foot. The swelling and redness spread over the foot, and the person can walk only with much suffering.

Attacks can be precipitated by acute or chronic injury to the foot, by dietary excesses or overindulgence in alcohol, and by surgical operations. Susceptible persons often have their first attack of gout while resting in bed recovering from a hernia, gallbladder or other operation. Most of the time the attack comes "out of the blue," and no provocative factors can be ascribed.

Fortunately, with treatment the acute arthritis of gout can disappear as rapidly as it comes on, and even without treatment the initial attack subsides over a period of several days to several weeks without any residual arthritis. The usual course is for later recurrences in the same or the other foot and then in other joints, especially the ankle, heel, and knee. Only one joint is involved at a time, as opposed to rheumatoid arthritis, where several joints are often symmetrically affected. Without proper treatment, recurrent attacks can leave the joints chronically painful, stiff, and enlarged. Serious deformities can even result. Many times uric acid is deposited in the tissues of the ear, over knuckles and other joints, and under the skin; these lumps, which are painless, are called tophi. They only occur when the blood uric acid has been high for many years. Much more seriously, uric acid is also laid down in the kidneys, and over long periods of time can slowly destroy the kidneys and even cause the death of the victim. Kidney stones of uric acid frequently occur.

If treated early, an attack of acute gouty arthritis will usually respond dramatically to an ancient drug called colchicine; the pain and swelling are often gone within 24 hours. It is said that Benjamin Franklin, a victim of gout, brought this remedy to America from Europe. Colchicine is less effective if the condition has existed for more than a very few days. In these cases either indomethacin (Indocin) or phenylbutazone (Butazolidine) is quite beneficial. Even after the painful, red, swollen joint has returned to normal, however, the patient still has his abnormally high blood level of uric acid. This must be corrected in order to prevent further attacks as well as to protect the kidneys from damage. Fortunately, this is easily done by means of medication. Two drugs are available that will maintain normal blood uric acid levels in persons with gout: probenecid (Benemid), which increases the amount of uric acid removed from the body in urine, and allopurinol (Zyloprim), which interferes with the chemical reaction whereby uric acid is produced.

Backaches and Disorders of the Spine
The subject of backache rings a familiar note to all of us. For most of us, a backache is usually self-limited and improves with rest. Persistence of back discomfort brings many persons to a physician or chiropractor seeking relief of pain.

Backaches may follow a day of increased activity, such as spring cleaning with lots of lifting or washing of windows. It may follow a long uncomfortable car ride or be present many mornings upon first awakening. What causes this particular vulnerability of our back?

The evolutionary ascent of our ancestors allowed man alone to assume an upright position and gait, thereby providing maximal utilization of our arms. Unfortunately, our back development has lagged behind and the shift of our center of gravity to the area of our lower back leaves us prone to back injury and backache. A brief review of anatomy is helpful to appreciate the origin of backaches and the complexity of our back.

The back consists of the spine, composed of square bones with projections called processes, the vertebral bones. Within the vertebral bone is an opening or canal in which the spinal cord lies protected from injury by its bony shield. Nerve projections, called peripheral nerves, come off at regular intervals from the spinal cord and travel through small openings in the vertebra called foramina. The peripheral nerves travel to the various muscles in our body, bringing the impulses from our brain through the paths in the spinal cord, and stimulating coordinated movements of our limbs. These same nerves carry messages from our skin, muscles, and deep tissue, which relay to our brain centers the various sensations: pain, numbness, temperature, touch, position, and vibration. In between the vertebral bones are round pads or discs, which serve as cushions. Various muscles connect to the vertebral bones by insertions called tendons. Muscles, when stimulated by nerve impulses, serve as pulleys, providing movement of the limbs, ribs, and diaphragm. Ligaments, strong fibrous attachments, link bones and parts of our bones to one another, providing additional strength and support to our spinal column.

If one looks at a skeleton, several details become obvious. The head rests on our neck formed by the cervical vertebrae, which project slightly forward. The neck rests on our shoulders and on the twelve thoracic vertebrae that form our backward-curved midback. The ribs arise from our thoracic vertebrae and form our thoracic cage, which serves to protect our vital organs, heart, and lungs. The lower back is formed by the five lumbar vertebrae, which again curve forward, producing a slight hollow in the area of the lower back. The sacrum forms the lowest part of the back and curves backward. The coccyx or "tail bone" is the terminal portion of the spine. These series of curves, forward in the neck, backward in the midback, and again forward in the lower back, produce a reverse S-shaped spine. (See illustration 12.)

Certain persons are born with or develop, by poor posture, accentuations of these curves. A *kyphosis* is a marked increase in the normal rounding or backward projection of the

The Spine

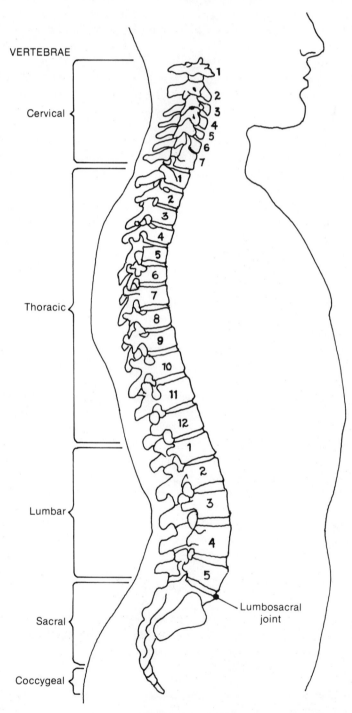

VERTEBRAE

Cervical

1
2
3
4
5
6
7

Thoracic

1
2
3
4
5
6
7
8
9
10
11
12

Lumbar

1
2
3
4
5

Lumbosacral
joint

Sacral

Coccygeal

Illustration 12

thoracic spine. An extreme example of this distortion of the spine is the famous Hunchback of Notre Dame. *Lordosis*, a pronounced curving forward of the lumbar spine, represents another type of back abnormality. In addition to the normal smooth curvatures of the spine forward or backward, the spine is usually straight or midline in its descent from the neck to the coccyx. *Scoliosis* is a curvature of the spine, neither backward nor forward, but sideways. A mild scoliosis is quite common, whereas a marked scoliosis produces a serious distortion of the body posture.

Backaches generally occur in the lower back where most of the stresses are felt. Disease, inflammation, or irritation of our muscles, nerves, discs, spinal cord, or ligaments may cause backaches. Similar inflammation or injury to the spine in the neck or upper back can cause pain and discomfort in these areas. Pain or discomfort is the final expression of various disorders of the lower back. The terms lumbago, low back syndrome, or strained back refer to poorly defined causes of back pain.

Low Back Syndrome. The most common cause of low back pain is injury and inflammation of the muscles of the back. Sometimes, no extraordinary physical activity may have occurred, but usually some vigorous activity has been performed a few days before the pain develops. Muscles that are required to support unusual activity levels are prone to be injured or strained by the excess effort. Most of us indulge in weekend activities that are strenuous compared to our regular pursuits. Several hours of gardening or snow shoveling or athletic exercise can cause a muscular strain. An irritated or strained muscle tends to contract or tighten and go into spasm. The pain gradually develops in the area of the inflamed muscles, the lower back, because of the contraction and shortening of the muscles and inability to relax and lengthen. If you flex your bicep muscle in your upper arm and maintain the contraction for several minutes, soreness and pain will develop.

At times, back muscles tighten and contract on account of injury to deep lying structures in the back such as ligaments or a ruptured disc. The pain associated with these processes causes reflex spasm of back muscles, further increasing the amount of pain.

Strained back muscles are common. Many people learn to live with them and reduce their activity level temporarily to avoid provoking discomfort.

If the discomfort persists, a physician may be consulted. Generally, a history of heavy lifting or some activity unusual for that individual is elicited. On examination, the inflamed or irritated muscles are prominent and the muscles are firm and contracted to the touch. The spine tends to list toward the injured side in an effort to relieve the contracted muscles. Efforts are made to exclude other disorders such as a herniated or ruptured disc. X-rays are seldom necessary.

Treatment involves avoidance of strenuous activities, bed rest on a firm mattress, and application of moist or dry heat, either hot towels or baths, or a heating pad. Aspirin is effective in control of pain. At times, stronger pain medicines may be necessary. Muscle relaxants may be quite effective in reducing spasm. Most muscle relaxants are sedatives and probably work by helping to encourage bed rest.

Often persons with chronic low back discomfort, especially present in the morning and disappearing during the day, incur back strain from sleeping on their stomach. The person who sleeps on his abdomen arches his back and causes irritation to his back muscles. This accounts for many morning backaches despite an otherwise comfortable sleep. Sleeping on the side or back corrects this problem.

Persons who are prone to backaches should try to strengthen their back muscles by exercises. Most physicians will describe exercises, called Williams' exercises, to achieve this end.

Discs. A disc is the cushion or pad that lies between adjacent vertebrae. The disc contains gelatinous material enclosed by a fibrous capsule. Rupture of the fibrous capsule allows for herniation or protrusion of the disc material, usually sideways, to impinge on nerve roots and cause symptoms.

A ruptured disc may occur at any level of the spine. The majority of disc ruptures occur in the lumbar area, so that low back pain is present. Usually the involved disc is between the fourth and fifth lumbar vertebrae or between the fifth lumbar vertebra and the sacrum. Disc problems also occur in the neck or cervical area and may impinge on the spinal cord itself, causing serious problems, including the possibility of paralysis.

A herniated disc in the lumbar area is quite painful and causes marked limitation of motion because of pain. Since the disc usually presses on nerve roots, pain of a shooting quality or a steady nagging pain which travels down the back of the leg to the knee or foot may be present. The pain is aggravated by coughing or sneezing. The person will move slowly when changing position to avoid pain. Often because of associated muscle spasm, the back muscles may be quite rigid. With involvement of the nerve roots, the usual ankle or knee jerk reflexes may be absent on the involved side. The physician looks for limitation of movement of the involved extremity, usually detected by an inability to elevate the leg to the same height as the other leg because of the onset of pain.

Disc problems may be treated by bed rest and analgesics, just as for a severe muscle strain. Traction, sustained pulling by weights placed on the involved extremity to help overcome muscle spasm and relieve pain, may be helpful, especially if the protruding disc slips away from the nerve roots. A myelogram is usually performed in a hospital for diagnosis of a ruptured disc. A spinal puncture is done, a needle introduced into the space surrounding the spinal cord, and a radio-opaque dye injected, which will show an indentation on the column of dye because of the herniated disc. Surgery is performed when symptoms of nerve compression do not respond to treatment. The irritation of nerve roots causes pain and numbness in the distribution of the peripheral nerve arising from the nerve roots. In addition, nerve injury leads to atrophy or shrinkage of the muscles supplied by the particular nerve.

Cervical discs, because of the location and possible pressure on the spinal cord, may require emergency surgery and decompression of the spinal cord to avoid permanent paralysis of the lower extremities.

"Whiplash" Injury of the Neck

This injury usually occurs during automobile collisions. The victim is sitting in an automobile, which is either traveling at a low speed or stopped when it is struck in the rear by another automobile. The victim's head is jarred forward or flexed and then pulled back or extended rapidly with sufficient force to injure muscles and other tissues of the neck. The neck muscles go into spasm, and pain in the back of the head and neck develops and becomes quite intense over several days. Treatments include the application of heat with hot water bottle or hot towels, pain killers such as aspirin, and muscle relaxants.

The Painful Shoulder

Of all the joints in the body, the shoulder is the most mobile. It is subject to a number of diseases which can cause pain, and this is a problem that frequently brings patients to the doctor. For reasons as yet unknown, the tendons around the shoulder joint tend to degenerate in middle-aged persons; when this happens, calcium is deposited in and around these tendons. Acute inflammation is a common complication. The resulting condition is called *calcific tendonitis.*

This usually begins suddenly with pain in the shoulder area, which may spread toward the neck or down the arm. The pain is severe and made worse by motion of the arm. The victim is unable to put his arm into his sleeve and indeed often unable to move the shoulder at all. The pain seems to be worse at night.

A similar pain seems to occur in *bursitis* at the shoulder. The subacromial bursa is a flat sac containing a tiny amount of fluid that overlies the tendons of the shoulder and normally serves to reduce the effect of friction when these tendons move. When the bursa becomes inflamed, it fills with more fluid. The resulting pain becomes extremely severe, and the victim will be afraid to move his arm. Putting the shoulder joint at rest and using anti-inflammatory medicines such as phenylbutazone and indomethacin frequently gives relief. When the condition is acute, injections of a local anesthetic (often in conjunction with a cortisone-like drug) may provide a rapid cure. Sometimes x-ray therapy is required for bursitis, and occasionally surgical removal of the calcium deposits is necessary for bursitis or tendonitis.

There are other causes of acute shoulder pain. Arthritis can involve the joint; the muscles and tendons can easily be torn; the tissues around the shoulder may become inflamed after a heart attack or stroke. Examination and x-ray study are necessary to make the proper diagnosis of the cause of a painful shoulder, so that correct treatment can be undertaken.

Sprained Ankle

A sprained ankle is extremely painful. This injury occurs usually when a person is running, but it may occur even in walking when the foot slips and is twisted inward, stretching and injuring the muscles and tissue around the outer ankle. The pain is instantaneous and severe, and the person is unable to bear weight on the foot and has to hobble or be carried.

If possible, an x-ray should be obtained to rule out a possible fracture. Treatment should consist of staying off the leg for 24 hours to 48 hours and, most importantly, application of cold compresses or ice to the area to minimize the painful soft tissue swelling that is caused by bleeding from injured blood vessels. The ankle and foot may be strapped in a day or so with an elastic bandage, and crutches may be required for five to ten days or longer until healing occurs. After the first day or two, soaking the foot in warm water helps to relieve discomfort and accelerate the reabsorption of blood and healing.

Symptoms you should know about:

Rheumatologic diseases usually cause **pain in the joints, bones, or muscles,** and frequently are responsible for **swelling of involved joints.** Other symptoms are **stiffness** and limitation of motion. Occasionally constitutional symptoms predominate, such as **fever,** or **weakness** due to anemia.

SKIN

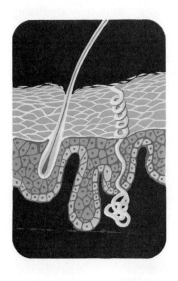

Although beauty is "only skin deep," our initial impression of people is certainly influenced by their overall appearance. How they look to us depends on their clothes, general body build, and facial features as well as the condition of their skin. The great concern people have for their skin and their efforts to alter, improve, or change it is reflected in the size of the cosmetics industry and the numbers of products and revenues generated. Even in ancient times and primitive cultures, dyes, paints, pigments, and various other preparations were applied to the skin for religious, cultural, and beautifying effects. In fact, many skin problems seen in any medical practice today are caused by the vast quantities of skin powders, lotions, detergents, deodorants, and cosmetics people apply to their skin, largely to enhance their appearance.

Skin serves the vital function of protecting our bodies from physical and chemical irritants in our environment. It is a tissue composed of cells, nerves, blood vessels, glands, and connective tissue. The *epidermis*, about as thick as this paper, contains cells that produce a skin protein called keratin, and a skin pigment called melanin. The epidermis lies on top of the *corium* or dermis, approximately twenty times the

195

thickness of the epidermis. The epidermis and dermis rest on subcutaneous tissue composed largely of connective tissue. Specialized forms of keratin form hair and nails. Sebaceous glands in the skin produce skin oils, and eccrine glands produce sweat.

Skin varies from one part of the body to another in thickness, suppleness, and gland content. The skin of our eyelids obviously differs from that of our soles and palms. Sweat glands are found in our palms and soles, whereas sebaceous glands are not; sebaceous glands are present in our earlobes but sweat glands are missing.

Skin also prevents loss of internal body fluids to the outside, helps maintain our internal temperature, and relays sensory information to the brain from nerve endings located in the skin. Skin diseases may involve disorders of the epidermis, hair and nails, sweat and sebaceous glands, or the dermis.

The epidermis contains two types of cells, the squamous or epidermoid cell, which produces keratin, and the melanocyte, which forms melanin. The content of the skin pigment, melanin, accounts for the color differences between light and dark complexions and the various races. Tanning from sun exposure is due to increased melanin production, which serves to protect the skin from damage by the ultraviolet rays of the sun.

Freckles are areas of the skin with a locally increased number of melanocytes. Skin moles, brown or black, are benign tumors or growths of melanocytes.

Sebaceous glands, oil producing glands, are most numerous in the scalp and forehead areas and drain into hair follicles. Blockage of gland ducts causes cysts to form. If bacteria penetrate the cyst, an infected, painful abscess results which can require surgical drainage and excision.

Sweat glands are involved in maintaining body temperature; evaporation of sweat cools the surface of the skin and aids in heat loss from the body. Modified sweat glands produce wax in the ear canals. Sweat is sterile and odorless but quickly becomes rancid, causing body odor because of bacterial contamination. Heat rash may occur by blockage of sweat glands due to injury or irritation to the skin such as a sunburn.

The skin itself may be involved in disorders such as poison ivy or psoriasis, or it may reflect internal derangements and diseases. Various skin rashes are seen with common viral infections, such as measles or chickenpox. Abnormalities of skin are sometimes seen in psychoneurotic illnesses, internal cancers, endocrine and hormonal problems, blood vessel diseases, connective tissue disorders, parasitic and fungal infections, various allergic conditions, and nutritional deficiencies. The skin mirrors our internal health; careful examination of it by physicians often suggests other disorders.

Skin Changes with Aging
Nowhere is the generalized aging that affects all body organs more apparent and distressing than in the skin. Man's perpetual search for a fountain of youth certainly applies to the great efforts many people expend in an attempt to preserve the beauty of their skin. Hours are spent in front of mirrors studying the skin appearance and applying cosmetics, skin lotions, and makeup to hide and cover the wrinkles, creases, and lines, moles, and other skin blemishes that develop with advancing age. The typical American bathroom cabinet contains numerous types of skin cosmetics used by women regularly in their homes. Visits to beauty salons for facial treatments are also common. The exploitation by the cosmetic industry of vanity applies to both sexes as more and more men have become concerned with their appearance.

As we age, our skin becomes thinner, less elastic, and rougher, reflecting the stresses and strains and wear and tear as well as hormonal changes occurring in many body organs. Exposure to the sun, winds, and other environmental factors causes the skin to be rough and wrinkled, an extreme example being a sailor or farmer working outside, whose facial skin may have the texture of parchment. The effects of weight gain, with stretching of the skin tissues, and weight loss, with loose and flabby skin, may be apparent. Skin aging is more noticeable in some people than in others. "Crow's feet" develop around the outer edges of the eyes, the skin of the lower eyelids becomes loose and flaccid, and the jowls sag.

Elderly people, whose skin is very fragile, bruise easily with minor trauma, especially on the upper arms. Such bruises are called *senile purpura*. Older people also tend to develop dry, itching skin, especially in winter, caused by a combination of decreased skin oils and the dryness of winter temperature and indoor heat. Under these conditions, too frequent bathing or washing of the skin aggravates the symptoms by further depleting the skin oil.

Hair, Baldness, and Hirsutism

The hair follicle is a tiny sac in the skin out of which the hair grows. There are about 100,000 hair follicles on the human scalp, each of which grows one hair at a rate of roughly one inch in 72 days. Although some persons have a much longer growth period, scalp hairs generally grow for about two to six years. They enter a resting period for several months, and then the hair is shed. A new hair begins to grow from the same follicle. Between 20 and 100 scalp hairs are lost every day, but these come from areas randomly scattered over the head, so their loss is not noticeable.

Hairs in areas of the body other than the scalp have different growth cycles, and in some areas (beard, armpits, body) are dependent on adrenal and testicular hormones for control of growth.

Male pattern baldness (common baldness) usually begins in the late 20s or early 30s with a gradual loss of hair, especially from the top and the front of the head. Eventually the entire scalp may become bald, or the sides and back of the head may be spared in the process. Premature alopecia (baldness) may begin in men in their early 20s. The cause of common baldness in men is unknown, but it seems to run in families.

Loss of hair, primarily involving the scalp, may also occur in hormone abnormalities due to disease of the endocrine glands, but is quite unusual. Sometimes hair loss is seen after a high fever. Certain drugs, especially those used in cancer chemotherapy, may cause temporary baldness.

Alopecia areata is the name of a condition in which the hair is lost in patches from the scalp. Its cause is unknown. If there are only a few patches of baldness, the outlook is good for regrowth and complete recovery. This occurs in about 80 percent of these cases in adults. Severe cases, especially in children, may involve most of the scalp, and the hair loss is frequently permanent. Certain curable fungal infections may cause patchy hair loss.

Alopecia totalis refers to loss of all the body's hair, including face, armpits, and pubic region.

There is no good treatment that will cause hair to grow in bald areas. In some cases of alopecia areata, cortisone injections into the scalp, or cortisone creams with plastic dressings seem to help regrowth of hair, but results are unpredictable. Nothing will produce hair growth in male pattern baldness. Transplantation of many tiny areas of hair-bearing skin to the bald scalp can be done, and sometimes quite acceptable cosmetic results are obtained.

Hirsutism means excessive amounts of hair, and this complaint is ordinarily confined to women who notice more hair than is acceptable in their culture. There are certain serious hormonal disorders that cause females to become virilized, that is, to develop a male appearance, with increased hair, lower voice, larger muscles, and other secondary characteristics of maleness. Occasionally other hormonal diseases can cause hirsutism without evidence of virilism. In women who are having regular menstrual periods and whose physical examination is normal other than the excessive hair, certain urinary tests may be done which will tell whether there is a hormonal disorder.

Most women who come to the doctor complaining of hirsutism do not have any definable hormonal disturbance. Exhaustive testing fails to reveal any abnormalities. In these cases the only available treatment is permanent destruction of the hair follicles by a process called electrolysis. Sometimes cosmetic techniques are useful in this problem.

Skin Tumors

In addition to changes in texture and wrinkling, which skin develops as part of the generalized process of aging, people develop various types of skin blemishes or lesions—moles, warts, and age spots—which cause concern. These growths are usually benign tumors, but malignant growths can also develop.

The common benign growths are seborrheic keratoses, senile keratoses, and fibromas.

Seborrheic keratosis usually develops in people with dark hair and brown eyes—dark complexion—who have oily skin. The growths are elevated, greasy, brown or black, and can fairly easily be scraped off the skin surface. They occur commonly on the face, back, and chest. They are not cancerous and are of little concern except for their appearance.

Senile keratosis tends to be flat, brown or tan in color, and firmly attached to the skin. The growths develop in people with light complexions, usually in sun-exposed areas of the skin—the face and back of the hands. They have the potential of becoming malignant and should be watched and removed if the growth increases rapidly.

Fibromas are individual or multiple skin tags on the neck or armpit areas, usually in middle-aged, overweight people. They are always benign and generally offer no problem. Removal is recommended only for cosmetic reasons and to avoid irritation from shirt collars or undergarments.

Malignant tumors develop in the epidermis. The most common malignant skin tumor is the *basal cell tumor*, which is 100 percent curable if treated early and adequately. These tumors do not metastasize or spread to other areas of the body and almost all develop on the face. Typically, basal cell tumors develop in fair-skinned people, in areas of sunlight exposure. The tumor begins as a small nodule, which gradually enlarges over a period of many months to form an area of central depression with a raised pearly border. There is a greater incidence in persons who have been exposed to facial x-ray or radium treatments. Surgical excision of the growth along with a margin of normal skin usually is curative. The specimen is reviewed by a pathologist to ensure that the margins of the removed growth contain no residual tumor; otherwise, a more radical excision must be done to ensure removal of all the tumor tissue. When such tumors occur on the face, x-ray treatment is often used in order to avoid scarring.

The *squamous cell tumor* is the other malignant growth arising from the epidermoid cell. This tumor may arise from any area of the skin but most commonly occurs on the lower lip, ears, tongue, and back of the hand. It can arise from a preexisting senile keratosis or begin de novo. Other possible causes include excessive sun exposure, radiation, chemicals, and mechanical trauma, such as pipe smoking. This tumor can spread to other areas of the body, commonly the lymph nodes. A high rate of cure can be achieved with early treatment by surgical excision, often combined with x-ray treatment to adjacent areas.

Melanocytes, the color-producing cells, can also form malignant tumors called *melanomas*. They arise from moles. Any sudden change in the color or size of a mole, an increase in pigmentation, or an irregular pigmentation, or bleeding or ulceration requires prompt medical evaluation. In general, moles with stiff hairs growing from them do not undergo malignant change. To relieve anxiety and concern about possible cancer, one should mention and show skin growths to the doctor, who can either allay one's fears or recommend excision of suspicious growths.

Acne Vulgaris

Acne vulgaris or acne is the common skin affliction of the adolescent. It is caused by excessive fatty acid secretion by oil-producing skin glands. Blockage of the oil gland duct leads to a blackhead, or comedone; an inflammatory reaction occurs and infection may develop, producing red pimples and painful deep cysts which may discharge their waxy material or slowly resolve, leaving scars.

Many teenagers develop mild acne, which is almost a stage of adolescence, producing little permanent damage or disfigurement, and which tends to disappear with age and perhaps improved skin care.

Acne seems to run in families, especially those with oily, greasy skin. It usually occurs on the forehead and face, neck, back, and chest. It is aggravated by poor skin hygiene and infrequent skin washing as well as the dietary disasters of the teenager. Nervous tension can aggravate the condition, and hormonal factors play a role. Acne generally begins at puberty and exacerbates in the female premenstrually.

The usual mild case of acne generally does not require evaluation by a physician. More serious, advanced cases should be seen by a physician or a skin specialist, a dermatologist. Untreated, acne cysts form scar tissue and leave pits or disfiguring pock marks on the skin.

The teenager has the already difficult challenge of making the transition from childhood to adulthood. Their bodies may be adult size, but emotionally they are still quite fragile and cannot accept any loss of self esteem caused by peer rejection. To be plagued with "zits and zorts" may subject the teenager to cruel teasing, prevent normal companionship, dating experiences, etc., and cause a sense of isolation and a feeling of inferiority.

Treatment of acne involves efforts to improve skin hygiene and to alter the diet by avoiding acne-provoking foods.

Since acne is caused by excessive skin oils, greasy or oily face lotions and salves should be avoided, and since it is often associated with dandruff and oily hair, greasy or oily hair tonics should also not be used. Careful washing of the involved areas of the skin three or four times a day, using soap and water, removes excessive oil. Special creams and soaps are available to cleanse and dry the skin.

An adequate diet is important, including fresh fruits, vegetables, and lean meat. Chocolate in any form—cake, ice cream, candy bars—as well as nuts should not be eaten. Greasy and fried foods should not be eaten (pizza, fried chicken, french fried potatoes, etc.). Whole milk, sharp cheeses, cream cheese, and whipped cream should be eliminated and replaced with skim milk and cottage cheese. Foods that contain iodine, such as iodized salt and ocean fish and shellfish, stimulate the oil-producing glands to increase oil production and should not be eaten.

Other general measures include adequate rest and avoidance of stressful situations. Sunlight in moderate exposure is good, for it helps dry the skin, but a sunburn should be avoided.

Recently, low dose, broad spectrum antibiotics, such as tetracycline, have been found effective in improving acne. For severe acne, close supervision by a dermatologist is in order. He may resort to treatment with ultraviolet light. Fortunately, 90 percent of adolescents will suffer no serious complications from their acne and respond to the measures outlined above.

Contact Dermatitis

One of the most common skin eruptions is contact dermatitis—an inflammatory skin reaction caused by an allergic response to an agent coming into contact with the skin.

The range of offending agents is large and includes paints, varnishes, lacquers, plants (including poison ivy, oak, and sumac), jewelry, foodstuffs, cleansers and detergents, insecticides, industrial chemicals, dyes, cosmetics, and clothing. Usually the rash does not occur upon first exposure but develops after many contacts with the agent. Certain substances sensitize most people who come into contact with them, whereas others sensitize only a small percentage.

Contact dermatitis involves all ages and races, and both sexes. Usually, in a mild case, redness and mild itching are the only symptoms. In a more serious case, swelling may develop with formation of blisters and crusts and weeping of fluid. Intense itching may lead to scratching and a secondary skin infection.

A common contact dermatitis is the reaction to the nickel that is present in costume jewelry, including earrings, rings, and watchbands. Such a localized rash clears when the offending jewelry is no longer worn. By similar detective work, other skin rashes caused by a vast array of potential agents can be identified. Dermatitis involving the eyelids alone or sides of the neck may be due to nail polish and the contact of the skin in these areas by the hands. A rash under the armpits may be caused by deodorants, and in women a rash and irritation in the groin area may be due to a feminine hygiene spray.

Most contact dermatitis occurs on the exposed parts of the body. The backs of the hands are involved in most occupational exposures and in the reaction to detergents commonly experienced by the housewife.

The treatment of this type of skin disorder involves identification of the cause and avoidance of the substance. Generally, a manufacturer removes a chemical or agent from the market if a significant percentage of those exposed develop such a skin reaction. In industry, protective garments, such as masks, gloves, or aprons, are provided to prevent contact with a potentially irritating substance. The housewife may wear rubber gloves in laundry work or dishwashing to avoid the reddened, rough, and itching skin that otherwise might result.

Poison Ivy (Oak or Sumac). Most of the patients with poison ivy dermatitis are children. As soon as contact with the plant is made, the skin on the exposed portions should be thoroughly washed with a bar of soap to remove as much of the plant oil as possible. Calamine lotion or other soothing anti-itching solutions should be applied to the skin. In widespread involvement, use of oral or intramuscular steroids is quite effective but requires close physician supervision. Patients who have shown a high degree of vulnerability to poison ivy should be considered for allergy shots to desensitize their skin early in the spring.

Learning to avoid contact with the plant by recognizing it as growing in clusters of three leaves is important.

Psoriasis

Psoriasis is a common skin disorder of unknown cause. The disease rarely affects infants or young children but develops during adolescence, reaching a peak incidence during mid-adulthood. A family history of psoriasis is often present.

The areas of the skin commonly involved include the scalp, the lower part of the back, the rectal and groin areas, and the pressure points around the knees and elbows. Any or all of the skin of the body may be involved. An extreme example of generalized psoriasis was the alligator man of the carnival sideshow, who was covered from head to toe. The affected areas usually are oval red patches or plaques covered by layers of silvery scales which shed regularly.

Psoriatic skin has an increased proliferation or production of cells so that more are being formed than in normal skin. The replacement of epidermis cells, which usually takes 28 days in normal skin, is reduced to 3 or 4 days in psoriasis because of this accelerated cell activity.

The nails may be involved in psoriasis, producing pitting and deformity as well as thickening. Psoriasis of the nails must be distinguished from fungal infections. Psoriasis of the scalp can be confused with seborrheic dermatitis. At times, an arthritis, usually of the hands and feet, can be associated with psoriasis and be quite deforming and disabling.

Psoriasis can develop in skin involved in minor trauma. Excess sunlight, scratches on the skin, or even adhesive tape can produce psoriatic patches.

Innumerable remedies have been tried in an effort to control the disease. Although the word psoriasis is derived from the Greek "psora," meaning itch, itching is usually not a serious problem. Treatments that are effective appear to be those that inhibit or decrease cell turnover in the epidermis.

Ultraviolet light and sunlight, in moderate exposure, can bring great improvement. Coal tar derivatives, often combined with salicylic acid to improve penetration of the skin, have been effective in some cases. Anthralin combined with zinc oxide paste is a common type in use.

Steroid creams or ointments applied to the involved areas are effective in removing the scales and improving the skin. Often occlusive dressings, such as plastic film (Saran Wrap) applied over the steroid ointment, improves the result.

Striking improvement with a drug effective in cancer treatment, methotrexate, has recently been achieved. However, many potential side effects on other body tissues, including the blood and liver, can develop, so that use of this drug by experienced physicians should be limited to those with widespread disease.

The course of psoriasis is chronic and unpredictable. Fortunately, the disease is generally confined to a few areas of the body. Spontaneous improvement as well as worsening of the condition may occur. The majority of patients can achieve satisfactory control with the measures discussed above.

Seborrheic Dermatitis

Seborrheic dermatitis includes dandruff of the scalp but can also affect the groin and axillas (armpits), as well as the skin around the sides of the nose, forehead, eyebrows, eyelids, and behind the ears. It is usually associated with excess oiliness of the skin, although no abnormality of the oil or sebum has been identified.

Seborrhea can begin in childhood and persist throughout life. The yellow waxy, adherent scalp scales of the infant cradle cap is a form of seborrheic dermatitis. The typical involved skin shows reddish raised skin with yellowish greasy scales on the forehead, ears, neck, and face.

The seborrheic disorders have a chronic course with exacerbations and remissions. Treatment involves medicated shampoos and soaps that contain combinations of sulfur, salicylic acid, and resorcinol. Selenium sulfide is also effective. The ideal agent, which would be free of any side effects, such as inducing allergy, requiring infrequent use to control the itching, scaling, and oiliness, and be cosmetically acceptable, has yet to be found.

Herpes Simplex (Cold Sores)

A virus called herpes simplex causes a very common problem—cold sores, or fever blisters. Most people have been exposed to the virus at some time. For some unknown reason, certain individuals develop recurrent crops of blisters or cold sores in their mouth or on their lips, often associated with upper respiratory viral infections and fever, dental manipulation, exposure to sunlight, or emotional stress.

Uncommonly, the virus can cause severe infection of the eye or the central nervous system. Two forms of this virus have been identified. Herpes simplex type I causes the painful cold sores of the mouth and lip area, usually infects above the waist, and is transmitted by oral contact. Herpes simplex type II usually occurs below the waist, commonly involves the genitalia, and is usually transmitted during sexual intercourse. There is an association between cancer of the cervix and infection with herpes simplex type II virus. Infection with genital herpes virus appears to be increasing in frequency.

The many different measures used to treat herpes simplex infection indicate the ineffectiveness of therapy for this disease. Treatment in the past has involved using various salves, ointments, and smallpox vaccination.

Recently, photoactive dyes have been shown to cause faster healing of the blisters and fewer recurrences. The virus can incorporate dyes, such as neutral red, and when the involved areas are exposed to fluorescent light for varying intervals the virus is inactivated.

Enthusiasm for phototherapy must be tempered by experimental evidence which suggests that viruses inactivated in this manner are able to induce cells to undergo malignant transformation; thus the photoactive dyes may subsequently increase the risk of cancer.

Fungal Infections

Fungi are microorganisms closely related to bacteria that can penetrate the skin and cause infection and inflammation. Commonly, the various species of fungus have a predilection for certain areas of the skin and cause specific clinical pictures. Involvement may be confined to the scalp, beard, the folds of the skin, the nails, hands, or feet (in this case producing the common disorder of athlete's foot).

Monilia, caused by the fungus Candida albicans, can involve the skin folds under the armpit, in the groin, under the breasts, or inside the mouth (thrush) or vagina. The affected skin is red, itchy, and scaly. Treatment is generally effective with an antifungal agent, nystatin, or gentian violet solutions.

Ringworm refers to the fungal infection of the smooth skin forming red, scaly, oval patches, which spread centrifugally leaving clear centers, often looking like concentric circles or bulls' eyes. Tolnaftate (Tinactin) cream or ointment applied to the involved areas usually eradicates the fungus.

Athlete's foot (needless to say, you do not have to be an athlete to develop this fungal disorder) can involve anyone, but occurs most frequently in young males. The fungus occurs most commonly in association with warm conditions and excess sweating. Since the fungus thrives in conditions of warmth, moisture, and darkness, the athlete with sweating, moist feet is a natural candidate for fungus infection. Most gymnasiums and locker rooms are reservoirs of the fungus, so that improper drying of feet and contact with floors, rugs, and shower stalls allows for exposure to it. Once the fungus develops, shoes, and especially sneakers and bedslippers, serve as a source of reexposure and reinfection, which explains why certain people continue to have fungal infections despite temporarily successful efforts to eradicate them.

Athlete's foot usually starts in the skin webs between toes, producing redness, swelling, and blistering, and eventually splits or fissures in the skin, which are quite painful and itchy. The fungus spreads to the sides of the feet and involves the soles of the feet. The nails are often affected and show thickening, yellow discoloration, brittleness, and even a lifting from the nail bed. Nail involvement alone has to be distinguished from other disorders, including psoriasis.

The treatment of athlete's foot depends to some extent on the degree of skin and nail involvement. Fungal infection of webs and sides of toes usually responds to undecylenic acid preparations, which are available as powders, ointments, or sprays. For extensive foot involvement, soaking the feet in potassium permanganate solution regularly over a period of weeks can be quite beneficial. Treatment of nail bed disease is more difficult, since eradication takes several months until new nail growth replaces the diseased portion of the nail. Griseofulvin, a drug effective against fungus infection of the nails, should be used only under a physician's supervision.

Symptoms you should know about:

Skin disease is usually obvious to the patient. Any **persistent rash, a sore that doesn't heal,** or **a mole that is enlarging or changing color** should be brought to the doctor's attention because prompt treatment may be necessary.

INFECTIOUS DISEASES

10

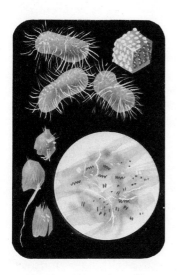

The history of medicine goes back thousands of years. Efforts at healing are as old as man, and every society has had some priest, healer, or medicine man who tried to end human disease and suffering by means of sacrifices, prayers, incantations, or with various herbs, compounds, or drugs. Although the roots of medicine are long, the major concepts of modern medicine have emerged within the past 100 years or so, with striking developments within the past 25 to 30 years.

The nineteenth century witnessed huge advances in the biological sciences. Schleiden and Schwann developed the cell theory of living organisms for plants and animals respectively. Darwin shook the world with his description of the evolution of species. The concept of inheritance and the science of genetics were developed by Mendel. Koch and Pasteur established the germ theory as the cause of many diseases—infectious diseases.

The remarkable extension of human life of about 30 years which has occurred in the United States from the turn of this century to our current decade represents largely a reduction in deaths caused by various infectious diseases that particularly strike the young. The changes in the vital statistics for the leading causes of death in this country for the period of

1900 to the present are striking. The three leading causes of death currently, heart disease, strokes, and cancer, were not even among the top ten causes of death in 1900, because childhood diseases led the list, and some that appeared in 1900 have been eliminated (diphtheria), or have largely been controlled (tuberculosis). (See Appendix I)

The branch of medicine that tries to prevent disease through application of new scientific knowledge and public information is called *preventive medicine*. In the area of many infectious diseases, effective methods for prevention have been achieved. When certain infectious diseases do occur, effective treatment is available with a list of antibiotics and other drugs that has been increasing since the introduction of sulfonamide in 1937.

Once it was recognized that many diseases were caused by germs (bacteria, viruses, rickettsiae, spirochetes, protozoa, fungi), often transmitted by vectors (carriers of disease from one person to another, such as certain mosquitoes, which can transmit malaria or yellow fever from one individual to another, or lice, which can spread typhus from person to person) or spread by using contaminated food and water, large-scale public health measures were instituted to protect the population.

Yellow fever, malaria, cholera, and typhoid fever have been almost entirely eliminated by public health measures at local, state, and federal levels to improve waste disposal and sanitation, rigid safeguards over our water supplies, and widespread use of insecticides to destroy the breeding areas of mosquitoes. Improvement of our standard of living—improved diets and home sanitation—has reduced transmission of infectious diseases as well as improved resistance to certain infections.

The widespread use of routine, mandatory vaccinations has prevented and eliminated many infectious diseases that formerly killed or debilitated thousands. Although smallpox vaccination was developed in 1798, routine vaccination for diphtheria, tetanus, pertussis (whooping cough), smallpox, measles, rubella (German measles), and poliomyelitis has largely eliminated these diseases as causes of human suffering and death in this century. Despite major advances in eradicating many infectious diseases, new ones are being recognized, such as "Legionnaire's Disease."

Immunization

Immunization, the process of developing resistance or immunity to various infectious diseases by using vaccines, is begun in infancy and continued through childhood when many potentially serious illnesses occur. There are two sorts of immunization, active and passive.

Active immunization consists of administering a biological product, usually by injection into the skin or, in the case of poliomyelitis immunization, taking it by mouth. The preparation called a *vaccine* (named after vaccina or cowpox, the first substance used in immunization by Edward Jenner to prevent smallpox) may be a live but weakened form of the germ such as is used for mumps, German measles, or poliomyelitis; it comes close to simulating a naturally acquired infection, thereby offering the most durable protection. Other types of vaccines are derived from killed or inactivated preparations of infectious agents. These include influenza and typhoid vaccinations. Toxoids are preparations of chemically altered products of bacteria called toxins, for example, diphtheria and tetanus toxoid. Vaccines induce the formation of antibodies in the person receiving them, and therefore afford protection or immunity for a variable period of time against the infectious agent.

Passive immunization is the giving of an antibody derived from a previously immunized animal or human, to a person who has not previously been immunized. This is done when the seriousness of the potential infection will not allow for the time it takes to form antibodies by active immunization. Examples include a rabies infection or tetanus infection.

Antibody levels induced by various vaccines tend to decline over a period of years and may be undetectable. Booster injections are necessary for diphtheria and tetanus at ten-year intervals, but adults do not require immunization with measles, pertussis (whooping cough), polio, or smallpox vaccines.

Travelers to foreign countries should check with their local Board of Health regarding current recommendations for vaccination against typhoid, cholera, typhus, plague and viral hepatitis.

The success in eliminating certain infectious diseases has permitted a relatively lax attitude toward continued immunization in the adult population, and many persons remain susceptible to two preventable diseases, diphtheria and tetanus. This neglect is unfortunate because immunization is safe, relatively inexpensive, easy to administer, and offers long-term, and in some cases permanent, protection against a variety of infectious agents.

A schedule of immunization is provided in Appendix II at the end of the book.

Temperature Controls

The maintenance of a relatively constant body temperature is an example of our nearly perfect internal controls. Our body temperature is usually maintained within one or two degrees Fahrenheit, despite the season of the year, the amount of clothing worn, and even the external temperature. This nearly perfect thermostat-like control is maintained by a temperature center in the brain. Yet there is nothing sacred about an oral temperature of 98.6 degrees Fahrenheit or a rectal temperature that is one degree higher. Often persons are concerned about a body temperature that is less or slightly more than 98.6. Very commonly, our temperature may be as low as 96 degrees or less, especially in the morning when we first awaken, and may be as high as 99.6 or even 100 in the latter part of the day. A woman's basal body temperature, that is, the temperature taken first thing in the morning before getting out of bed, is lower during the first half of her menstrual cycle. When ovulation occurs, halfway through the cycle, the basal temperature goes up a small amount.

Skin Temperature.   In normal health, the body temperature remains fairly constant. Heat is a normal byproduct of our body machinery and must somehow be disposed of. Heat loss largely occurs by conduction, whereby heat moves from a warm surface to a cooler one (as in our home radiators). If the body needs to conserve heat and minimize heat loss through conduction, blood is directed away from the skin and shunted through deeper-lying blood vessels. If heat loss is necessary, blood vessels on the skin become dilated and blood flow is increased, promoting heat loss by conduction. Naturally, skin with a lot of blood flow through it feels warm and skin with minimal blood flow feels cool to the touch.

When we exercise, our faces may become flushed and our bodies warm, facilitating heat loss. Our body temperature, as felt in warm or cool hands and feet, is largely due to the body's attempt to conserve or lose heat.

Young or middle-aged women often mention that their feet

are so cold at night that their husbands complain about them. They are concerned that their "circulation" might be poor. Usually, however, the doctor finds the circulation, namely arterial pulses in the feet, to be quite good, and the coolness of the extremities is simply due to shunting of blood away from the skin to control heat loss.

Sweating. Sweating is another mechanism that allows heat loss. If the body temperature is similar to or less than that of the environment, heat loss cannot occur by conduction. In warm weather and in tropical areas, the evaporation of sweat from the body surface causes heat loss.

Sweat glands are scattered throughout the body, with large numbers located in the axillas (armpits) and on the forehead. Some persons have few or no sweat glands, and there are racial differences in the concentration of sweat glands in various areas of the body. When we are in a warm environment, within a few minutes beads of sweat start to form all over our skin, but they are most noticeable on the forehead, upper lip, neck, and chest. This is different from the pattern of sweating caused by anxiety and fear, when even in a cold atmosphere we break out in sweat, especially on the palms of the hands and in the armpits. Tense persons often complain of constant excessive perspiration of those areas.

Fever. Changes in body temperature often reflect associated disease processes. Very low temperatures may be seen in thyroid disease, when the thyroid is underactive. Elevated temperatures may be seen with certain malignant tumors, an overactive thyroid, or in many infectious illnesses. Indeed, fever is the hallmark of acute infections.

The temperature elevation or fever in an infectious disease, such as a viral illness like flu, or a bacterial pneumonia may in fact represent the body's attempt to overcome the offending organism. Fever in an adult is generally not harmful, if it is lower than 105 or 106 degrees Fahrenheit.

In young children, a fever may be associated with seizures or convulsions and is, therefore, more serious. Vigorous efforts to restore the temperature to normal, usually by large amounts of aspirin, should be discouraged, except in young children. Sponge baths, especially with alcohol, are helpful.

The Common Cold and Influenza
Colds are upper respiratory infections caused by certain viruses that produce illnesses that are highly contagious but

nonfatal. The pattern of a cold varies according to the particular strain of virus as well as differences in the patient. Generally, the sinuses are congested and the nose alternately stuffy and running. A cough may be present, along with low grade fever, weakness, and headache, and there are often gastrointestinal complaints, such as diarrhea. Certain viruses produce flu-like symptoms with muscle aching and high temperatures. Upper respiratory infections usually last five to ten days.

Despite the general impression that colds come from exposure to drafts or changes in temperature, there is little scientific evidence that this is true. Colds are caught by contact with people who are sneezing or coughing and thereby disseminating their viruses into the air and subsequently the nasal passages of others. Colds are, therefore, prevalent in school children, and they occur in adults who go into public places, such as markets, churches, or movie theaters. The average person has approximately three colds a year, although this may decrease in frequency in adult life. Viral infections stimulate antibodies to the particular virus strains, but dozens of viruses and strains exist and protection is not provided by antibodies to one strain against other strains of viruses. However, an upper respiratory infection often causes a relative resistance to another virus because of production of interferon, an antiviral factor, by the body following a recent upper respiratory infection.

Antibiotics are ineffective in the treatment of colds and are contraindicated for several reasons. All drugs are potentially harmful, and if no benefit is to be derived from them, they should not be used. Penicillin has no effect against the cold or other upper respiratory infection. Furthermore, it is possible to develop an allergy to an antibiotic by frequent use of a drug, so that it cannot be taken when it is needed, as for bacterial infection. Antibiotics often produce unpleasant side effects, such as diarrhea, and may allow for a superimposed infection by eliminating relatively harmless bacteria and allowing dangerous ones to flourish.

There is no effective treatment for colds other than supportive treatment, which means treating the symptoms that occur as part of the viral illness. Aspirin is effective for controlling muscle pain, aching of joints, headaches, and fever. Stuffy nose and postnasal drip often respond to antihistamines. Cough syrups are effective in controlling cough. Cold symptoms improve with rest.

Certain types of patients are more likely to develop complications of an upper respiratory infection. Smokers and persons who have chronic lung disease or bronchitis or emphysema are more likely to develop pneumonia (viral or more commonly bacterial) following a cold, or have an exacerbation of their chronic lung disease. Also in cigarette smokers colds often last longer than those of the nonsmoker. Elderly patients or patients with chronic illnesses are more likely to develop debilitating illnesses following a viral infection and should promptly receive medical attention.

Despite our increasing knowledge in medicine, effective prevention or modification of colds or upper respiratory infections eludes us. There is no good scientific evidence that vitamin C in any way prevents viruses or upper respiratory infections. Flu vaccinations provide fairly good protection against a specific virus, influenza, and usually against several strains. Such vaccinations are not 100 percent effective, and the antibodies produced by the flu shots do not protect against the many other viral agents that in fact cause the majority of upper respiratory infections. The newer preparations of the flu vaccine have been purified so they no longer produce unpleasant side effects, which in fact were a modified form of the flu. Generally, flu vaccination is indicated only in the elderly or in those with complicating illnesses, such as heart or lung disease.

Tuberculosis

Tuberculosis is caused by a bacterial organism called *Mycobacterium tuberculosis*, or the *tubercle bacillus*. At one time tuberculosis was the leading cause of death in America. The devastation caused by this infectious disease can be appreciated by its toll—more people have died from tuberculosis than in all wars in the history of the United States. The decline in the yearly death rate from 200 per 100,000 population in 1906 to 2.1 per 100,000 in 1971 reflects the overall improvement in hygiene, diet, and standard of living in this country as well as earlier recognition of the disease and effective drug treatment programs.

Although any organ of the body may be infected, the lungs are usually the main site. An infected person transmits infected droplets into the air when coughing or sneezing. The bacteria can survive for long periods in the air, and the organism has even been shown to be alive in the tombs of

Egyptian mummies thousands of years later.

Tuberculosis (TB) used to be acquired through drinking contaminated milk from infected cows, but bovine TB has now been eliminated in this country. In other countries, pasteurization of milk destroys any tubercle bacilli.

The initial exposure to tuberculosis produces *primary tuberculosis*. The person (often a child) with no previous exposure to the germ inhales the bacteria, which go into his lung during breathing. The body has no resistance to this organism, since it has never experienced it. The bacteria multiply in the lung and travel to lymph glands draining that area of lung, where they proliferate and can even reach the blood stream and travel to various body organs. After several weeks, resistance to this foreign agent develops, mediated by various cells in the area, including lymphocytes and macrophages. A vigorous body defense leads to resolution of the infection, finally producing a healed focus of scar tissue, which often calcifies.

Evidence to suggest previous exposure to tuberculosis can be obtained from a chest x-ray, which shows the scarring and calcification. Such changes, although most often due to TB, may also be the result of previous exposure to other infectious agents and are therefore not diagnostic of previous tuberculosis.

Once a person has been exposed to tuberculosis (the disease produces firm nodules or tubercles, hence its name), a positive skin reaction develops in response to an inoculation of a derivative of the killed tubercle bacillus. Several different tuberculin skin tests are available, including P.P.D. (purified protein derivative) and the tine test. An area of swelling or induration (like a mosquito bite) develops within 48 to 72 hours if a person has had previous exposure to the germ and is a positive reactor.

Approximately 30 percent of the population over the age of 50 react positively to tuberculin skin test, whereas only 3 to 5 percent of young adults have positive reactions, indicating the decrease in exposure and subclinical infections.

The majority of persons exposed to tuberculosis are able to mount a successful attack against this infectious disease and develop "healed" or dormant tuberculosis—recognized by the positive skin test and changes on a chest x-ray. Many of them cannot recall an episode during their lives when an illness that would account for their dormant TB occurred.

However, it is this reservoir of dormant or latent disease that largely accounts for the majority of cases of adult tuberculosis. The defense mechanisms that have effectively prevented progression of the disease break down, usually in association with other debilitating processes, such as alcoholism, chronic disease, malignancy, diabetes mellitus, or use of various drugs including corticosteriods. Reactivation of previous foci of tuberculosis, and not re-exposure, accounts for most cases of adult or *secondary tuberculosis*.

The symptoms of active tuberculosis include persistent fever, night sweats, chills, weight loss, and general malaise. Most symptoms are pulmonary and include cough, sputum production (phlegm), and even coughing up of blood. The chest x-ray is abnormal. The disease can involve other organs of the body, including the brain, kidneys, liver, and bone.

The diagnosis of active tuberculosis requires establishing the presence of the bacillus Mycobacterium tuberculosis. With special staining, phlegm from the person should show the presence of the bacteria. The sputum is submitted to a laboratory for culture, and after several weeks the organism grows, confirming the disease.

Treatment. The treatment of tuberculosis has changed dramatically in the past 25 years. What was once a hopeless disease, with patients confined for years in sanitoriums, eventually to die, can now be cured, and the prospect for elimination of this disease from this country is a real one.

Patients with active tuberculosis are initially confined to a hospital where treatment with two or three drugs is begun. Modern treatment reduces the infectiousness of the patient after several weeks, so prolonged hospitalization is no longer necessary.

The drugs usually selected include isoniazid (INH), combined with para-aminosalicylic acid (PAS) or ethambutol or rifampin. Another available drug is streptomycin, which is given by injection.

Treatment continues for 18 to 24 months. The patient is checked regularly, and sputum is examined to determine when organisms are no longer present. Once the cultures are negative on three consecutive tests, monitoring can be less frequent. Chest x-rays are obtained to document healing of the diseased areas of the lung, and follow-up x-rays are made for many years to ensure that treatment has been successful.

Surgical intervention, once a very important factor in the

management of tuberculosis before the availability of effective drugs, is now seldom necessary.

Finally, a vaccine called BCG, made from a live but weakened strain of bovine tuberculosis, reduces susceptibility to infection by about 80 percent. Its use is advocated in countries where many cases of the disease develop. It is not used frequently in this country except for persons with high risk of exposure (health workers) or among certain ethnic groups where disease is quite prevalent and their resistance to it is low (Eskimos). Opponents to its wide use cite the decreasing incidence of tuberculosis in this country and, since inoculation with the vaccine causes a positive skin test to tuberculin, the loss of this valuable sign as an indicator of recent exposure to tuberculosis.

Viral Hepatitis

Inflammation of the liver, or hepatitis, commonly occurs because of viral infections. Many different viral and presumed viral agents can cause liver injury or hepatitis, including yellow fever, cytomegalic inclusion disease, and infectious mononucleosis, to name a few. Hepatitis also can occur from noninfectious causes, including exposure to chemicals (for example, carbon tetrachloride), unusual sensitivity to drugs (isoniazid), or an anesthetic agent (halothane), and from excessive use of alcohol.

Two distinct types of the disease have been established on the basis of different incubation periods (the time between exposure and the symptoms and signs of the illness developing) as well as the way the disease is caught: *infectious hepatitis* and *serum hepatitis*. The former usually is transmitted from contamination of food via the oral route, with a period of two to six weeks before illness develops. Serum hepatitis generally is transmitted by an injection, such as a blood transfusion, or, in many cases, from needles used and shared by drug addicts. Hepatitis usually develops six weeks to six months later.

In general, what has been called infectious hepatitis may occur sporadically or as an epidemic with a high attack rate in a susceptible population, especially children. Crowded conditions and poor sanitation account for the high rates observed in institutions, such as hospitals for retarded children. Contamination of shellfish by polluted coastal waters has accounted for recent epidemics in the United States and for closure of areas for collection of shellfish. Recently, an out-break of infectious hepatitis affected an entire college football team due to contamination of drinking water. Although all the team had evidence on blood testing for hepatitis, some had minimal symptoms and were not jaundiced.

Serum hepatitis, transmitted from blood derivatives, has been reported from tatoo instruments, inadequately sterilized syringes and needles, and in persons who require frequent transfusions with blood derivatives. Hemophiliacs, who require factor VIII, a clotting factor derived from blood, as well as health workers who work in kidney dialysis units, have developed hepatitis. This kind of hepatitis has decreased considerably since techniques have become routine for detect-ing potential blood donors who harbor an antigen or marker identifying the presumed hepatitis virus. The Australian anti-gen, probably derived from a portion of the virus, first detected in the blood of an Australian aborigine, allows identification of blood donors who can transmit hepatitis.

Recently, evidence has developed that the division of the disease into two clinical patterns may be artificial. Serum hepatitis may also be transmitted through ingestion of con-taminated material, and the separation by incubation period may also not be as absolute as previously thought. In fact the presumed virus has never been successfully isolated in tissue culture and several different agents may be responsible for this illness. The symptoms and signs of hepatitis are generally divided into those that precede the onset of jaundice and those that accompany jaundice. However, many persons who develop hepatitis do not become jaundiced, and the disease may only be suspected and diagnosis confirmed by blood tests. As mentioned above, during an epidemic, cases are discovered because of possible exposure, vague symptoms, and subsequently the indication by blood tests of liver cell injury.

Symptoms prior to the onset of jaundice may be nonspecific and vague. A loss of appetite, fever, muscle and joint aching, weakness, malaise, headache, and nonspecific gastrointestinal complaints may be present from one to several weeks before the onset of jaundice. With the development of jaundice, that is, yellowing of the eyes and skin, fever usually subsides, and the liver is noted to be enlarged and tender. Generally the jaundice peaks within two weeks and goes away in several weeks.

For the vast majority of patients, hepatitis leaves no permanent injury to the liver and many cases are not even detected. Chemical evidence of the inflammation of the liver monitored from blood tests improves and returns to normal over several weeks or months. Fatigue and decreased stamina may remain for several months.

A small number (less than 1 percent of hospitalized patients) of those with clinical evidence of disease develop a more serious form of hepatitis with massive, progressive liver injury leading to death. In some, hepatitis may persist for long periods and progress to a chronic form eventually leading to fibrosis or scarring of the liver called *cirrhosis* (described in Chapter 4).

There is no effective treatment for viral hepatitis. Vigorous efforts are made to prevent spreading of the illness from bed linens and utensils used by the hepatitis patient. Bedrest may be helpful, but has not been proved to be associated with speed of improvement in young military personnel. An adequate and nutritious diet is important.

Screening of blood donors and eliminating blood containing Australian antigen have helped prevent serum hepatitis. Injections of gamma globulin are given to exposed persons to prevent the illness or make it less severe. Although jaundice does not develop, liver inflammation still occurs. More specific hyperimmune gamma globulin may significantly modify hepatitis transmitted by injection.

Venereal Disease
Venereal disease, which is infectious, is spread during sexual relations, and is a growing public health problem. When penicillin was discovered to be effective against syphilis and gonorrhea, a temporary decline in the incidence of these diseases gave some hope that they would join the list of infectious diseases that would no longer be a public menace. However, these expectations were not realized and rather than decreasing, they have become more frequent and more widespread. In addition to these two diseases, there is increased recognition of herpes simplex type II virus as a cause of transmissible venereal disease. Scabies and Pediculosis pubis (crab louse) are two other infectious diseases commonly spread by sexual contact that cause intense itching and a rash. Effective treatment is readily available when diagnosed. Contributing to the overall increase in venereal infections has

been the decline in the use of the condom as an effective birth-control device, which also cuts down on the transmission of infection between sexual partners.

Syphilis and gonorrhea continue to be a major public health concern. Teenagers and adults less than 25 years of age account for more than 50 percent of all cases of syphilis. It is estimated conservatively that 1.5 million new cases of gonorrhea occur annually.

The inability of public health officials to secure information from physicians and often the reluctance of persons with venereal disease to expose their contacts prevent proper identification of people who might have the disease. This latter group, most often unknowingly, serve as reservoirs of infection and continue to spread infection to unsuspecting contacts and perpetuate the disease in the community. Particularly in females with gonorrhea, symptoms and signs of venereal disease are often not present and no medical attention is sought.

A survey of physicians indicated that 80 percent of all cases of syphilis were treated by private physicians, who reported only 12 percent of cases to public health authorities. Two other less well known venereal diseases are lymphogranuloma venereum and granuloma inguinale. It is not uncommon for a person to develop more than one venereal disease at a time.

Syphilis. Sir William Osler said, "To know syphilis is to know medicine." Smallpox, the dread disease of the middle ages, which has been eradicated in the Western countries, was given its name to distinguish it from the "great pox," or syphilis.

Medical historians have argued for centuries about the origin of syphilis. One view is that it is an ancient disease, which has existed among civilized people for thousands of years. The other view argues that a particularly severe form or virulent disease spread across Western Europe shortly after Columbus returned from the New World. It was then introduced by Spanish mercenaries fighting with the armies of Charles VIII and spread throughout Italy. For a long time, other venereal diseases including gonorrhea were not distinguished from syphilis.

Syphilis is caused by an organism, *Treponema pallidum,* which requires the kind of warmth and moisture supplied by the body. It quickly dies outside of the body. The disease is transmitted through sexual relations. Despite general opinion to the contrary, one does not catch the disease from toilet seats, door handles, or drinking fountains.

There are four stages of syphilis. After exposure, no symptoms or signs of the disease develop for about three weeks (10 to 60 days), the incubation period.

The primary lesion or *chancre* develops at the site of inoculation, usually in the genital area, although mouth to genital contact permits the chancre to develop on the tongue, mouth, or lip area, and the anal area may also be involved, especially among homosexuals. The typical chancre or sore appears as a small erosion or ulcer and is usually painless. There is nothing absolutely characteristic of the appearance of a chancre that allows for an accurate diagnosis of syphilis. Only identification of the organism from scrapings of the chancre under a special microscope—one with a dark field mechanism—establishes the sore as a syphilitic chancre.

The chancre lasts several weeks and then disappears. The next phase of syphilis, *secondary syphilis*, is associated with mild symptoms, including general malaise and low grade fever, and a generalized body rash, which also affects the mucous membranes (mouth and genital areas) as well as the skin of the palms and soles. The rash usually lasts several weeks before it recedes, but it may recur for several months up to two years, until the body develops an acquired resistance to the organisms.

Latent syphilis, arbitrarily divided into early, less than two years from the original infection, to late latent, more than two to four years after the chancre, has no symptoms or signs.

Syphilis is very contagious or infectious during the primary and secondary stages. A small number of untreated persons with syphilis go on to develop late manifestations of syphilis, (*tertiary syphilis*) 15 to 20 years later, with involvement of the central nervous system (brain or spinal cord) or the cardiovascular system. Even if the disease is untreated, the body's defense mechanism controls the organism quite well. Syphilis proved to be the cause of death in 15 percent of males and 8 percent of females who had the disease but were not treated in a large study from Oslo, Norway.

Syphilis can be diagnosed by finding antibodies to the syphilis organism in the blood. The Wasserman test for antibodies was developed in 1906, followed by many others that were more specific and could be performed more rapidly. The VDRL test, an often-used serology test, becomes positive one to two weeks after the primary lesion or chancre forms, is always positive during the secondary phase, and remains positive during the latent stage. At times, a positive serological test can occur because of other diseases and is called a biological false positive test.

State laws require serology tests for syphilis for persons obtaining a marriage license. Tests are also performed routinely during pregnancy, since a mother with syphilis can introduce the infection to her fetus and cause either a stillbirth or syphilis in the newborn, which is called *congenital syphilis*.

Penicillin is almost 100 percent effective in treating syphilis. Patients treated early often revert to a negative blood test. The longer the disease exists before treatment, and if it becomes latent, the less likely is it that the antibody detected by a blood test will disappear altogether, but the level of antibody, called the titer, should either remain stable or decline. Periodic blood tests to measure the titer are performed to make sure additional treatment with penicillin is not needed. Late syphilis with evidence of brain or heart involvement requires special treatment.

Those allergic to penicillin can be treated with other antibiotics.

The control of syphilis requires the identification of all contacts of the known case. Since up to three months may have elapsed between exposure and the onset of the disease, all persons at risk during this interval should be interviewed and a blood test performed to ensure proper therapy.

Gonorrhea. Although gonorrhea may have been described in the Old Testament, it was not until the middle of the nineteenth century that the disease was clearly distinguished from syphilis. The misconception that gonorrhea was a symptom of syphilis was perpetuated by the famous physician John Hunter, who inoculated himself with pus from a person with gonorrhea who also had syphilis, and developed both diseases.

Gonorrhea, also known as the "clap," is caused by bacteria that infect the mucous membranes of the genital tract, and is transmitted during sexual relations.

In the male, approximately five to eight days after exposure, pain on urination and a discharge from the urethra develop. Without treatment, the discharge gradually decreases but a narrowing of the urethra may result from repeated attacks.

In the female, burning may occur upon urination, but the discharge often is small and not noticed. The infection can spread to the fallopian tubes and cause fever and pain in a condition called acute pelvic inflammatory disease. Blockage of the tubes may result in sterility. At times, acute gonorrhea can cause inflammation of joints producing an acute arthritis.

The frequency of gonorrhea is quite high. The carrier state, where a person harbors the bacteria but is free of symptoms, has been recognized more and more, even among males. Identification of asymptomatic contacts of persons who have had gonorrhea has established a relatively high percentage of asymptomatic carriers. The organism can be isolated and grown on particular culture media. Not only may the organism be present in the genital areas, but positive cultures can be obtained from the anal and oral areas as well, especially among homosexuals.

Gonorrhea is quite prevalent among servicemen who are stationed all over the world. Strains of gonorrhea, especially from Southeast Asia, are appearing that are less sensitive to penicillin and require larger doses of the drug.

Since the asymptomatic carrier state is recognized more and more, frequent bacterial cultures from the vaginal, urethral, oral, and anal areas of persons with wide sexual contacts will be necessary to identify and treat the reservoirs of this infection in our community in order to eradicate this disease.

Symptoms you should know about:

Fever is the hallmark symptom of infectious diseases, and is discussed in this chapter. However, some infections, even serious ones, may not be associated with fever. Other symptoms of infectious disease depend on the location, type of organism causing the disease, extent of involvement, and suddenness or slowness of the process. In general, a temperature over 101°F in adults or over 102°F in children should prompt a call to the doctor.

BLOOD

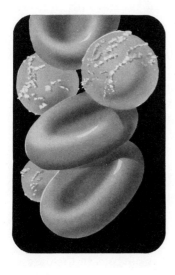

11

Television commercials and newspaper ads commonly warn us of anemia or too few red cells, and promote various medications and vitamins to regain our lost vitality and youthful energy. The "tired blood" of television ads a few years ago has become a household expression. Patients are told by their physicians that they have low blood pressure and assume vitamins are needed. Tiredness and lack of energy, very common complaints, are often believed by the patients to result from anemia due to lack of vitamins and iron. This chapter will tell you about the components and some of the disorders of the blood, as well as the relation of iron and vitamins to normal blood.

Blood is composed of a fluid layer, or plasma, and a cellular component containing three types of cells, which are manufactured in the marrow of bones: 1. red blood cells, 2. white blood cells, 3. platelets.

Red Blood Cells

The red blood cells (technically called erythrocytes) bring oxygen to the tissues of the body, which is the source of energy for many of the body functions. The oxygen is carried by a special protein in the red cells called *hemoglobin*. Red

225

cells survive for 120 days, so that approximately 0.8 percent of all our red cells must be replaced by our body everyday. A cubic millimeter of blood (the volume of a cube 1/25 of an inch on each side) contains about 5 million red blood cells. *Anemia* refers to an abnormal decrease in the number of red cells in the blood or in the amount of hemoglobin.

Anemia

The chief symptom of a person with significant anemia is tiredness. However, tiredness or lack of pep is often caused by other problems such as boredom, frustration, and, more often, mild depressive states. Other symptoms the anemic patient may complain of include shortness of breath with minimal exertion, dizziness, especially on rapid change of bodily position, and weakness. The anemic patient often appears pale and may have a rapid pulse. Whether anemia occurs within hours, such as following brisk bleeding, or in days or weeks, determines its symptoms. When the anemia develops slowly rather than quickly, the body is better able to cope with it.

There are three main reasons for anemia. The most common is a lack of raw materials needed by the factory, the bone marrow, to assemble red cells. Sometimes the factory itself is unable to manufacture red cells despite an abundance of raw materials. Finally, anemia can develop if there is increased loss or destruction of red cells in the body so that the factory is unable to speed up production to compensate adequately.

Lack of Raw Materials. The most common cause of anemia is iron deficiency. A small amount of iron is lost every day by the body. This loss is seldom significant except in the case of women, who need approximately twice as much iron daily as men do because of the blood loss accompanying the menstrual period. In addition, each pregnancy requires the mother's body to provide large amounts of iron for the developing fetus, and the delivery also causes a loss of some iron because of blood loss. Bleeding from any source causes a loss of iron. Therefore, iron deficiency can occur from a bleeding ulcer or any other disease in the gastrointestinal tract that causes blood to be lost, such as polyps or tumors. A pint of blood lost from the body removes approximately 250 mg. of iron. Normally, a man loses one milligram of iron every day and a woman an average of 2 mg. per day. Generally, iron deficiency in a young man is caused by gastrointestinal disease such as bleeding ulcers; in a woman of childbearing age because of heavy periods; and in older patients we have to consider cancer of the stomach or large bowel. Ulcers, polyps, or diverticuli are also causes of iron deficiency in any age group.

A fairly common cause of iron deficiency is the use of aspirin. Aspirin is an excellent drug for controlling pain and relieving inflammation and is used for headaches, joint and bone aches, and muscle soreness as well as many other conditions. However, it is quite irritating to the stomach and can cause erosion of the lining of the stomach, resulting in blood loss. Aspirin is present in many commonly sold drugs, but especially in pain pills, and this danger applies to all drugs containing aspirin, even the "buffered" types.

Iron is found in many types of food and is readily absorbed in the small bowel. Normally, the average American eating two to three meals per day will take in more than adequate amounts of iron for body needs, and less than 10 percent of the dietary iron is absorbed from his intestines. When iron deficiency develops, the body attempts to compensate by absorbing greater percentages of the iron available in the gastrointestinal tract. Several categories of patients are at risk for developing iron deficiency anemia. Infants and young children who consume milk, and are poor eaters otherwise, may develop iron deficiency, because milk is a poor source of iron. These children may appear healthy except for paleness. Women with heavy periods and who have had several pregnancies in close succession may become iron deficient. Persons who have had part of their stomachs removed, usually because of ulcers, are liable to develop iron deficiency because of poor absorption of iron in the gastrointestinal tract.

Iron deficiency can be corrected by iron-containing pills. The most effective form is ferrous sulfate tablets which contain approximately 90 mg. of iron. Iron pills will make the bowel movements darker in color. Some persons may become nauseated by iron preparations or complain of constipation.

Iron tablets should be taken only after the physician has obtained laboratory studies documenting the presence of anemia and other laboratory tests to detect the cause. The red cells that are present during iron deficiency are smaller and also appear pale under the microscope. Rarely, in certain susceptible patients, too much iron may be absorbed by the body because of a lack of regulation of iron absorption in the small bowel, and this may lead to iron overload in the tissues producing a disorder called hemochromatosis. This is why nutritionists are debating the merits of fortifying wheat and bread products with increased amounts of iron. Since iron tablets are one of the leading causes of childhood poisoning, such tablets, like all medications, must be securely placed away from a child's reach.

Another raw material needed to produce red cells is *folic acid*, a B-complex vitamin. Folic acid is found in meat and vegetables, and dietary lack is seldom a cause of anemia for the average person. However, several categories of persons may become deficient in folic acid and develop a significant anemia. Persons consuming large amounts of alcohol and otherwise eating poorly may develop folic acid deficiency. Elderly patients subsisting on a tea and toast type of diet may also become deficient in folic acid. This deficiency sometimes occurs during pregnancy, when the expectant mother may eat poorly. Patients who are chronically ill and hospitalized may develop folic acid deficiency, especially if they are receiving intravenous fluids as their main source of nutrition. A rare cause of folic acid deficiency occurs in infants fed goat's milk, which has little folic acid. Folic acid deficiency produces characteristic changes in the size and shape of red cells, and is readily suspected by the doctor from examining the blood smear. Folic acid deficiency can be effectively treated with vitamins containing folic acid.

Vitamin B_{12} deficiency is another cause of anemia, which is almost never due to dietary deficiency. *Pernicious anemia* occurs in a group of patients, generally older persons, who cease to manufacture in their stomachs a protein called intrinsic factor, which is necessary to allow vitamin B_{12} absorption by the small bowel into the body. The stomach fails to produce acid in this condition. The anemia develops quite slowly, but the lack of vitamin B_{12} in time causes damage to the brain and spinal cord. Vitamin B_{12} deficiency can be suspected by the typical changes of the blood smear, the findings in marrow material aspirated from the bone (from the hip or breastbone), and the low levels of vitamin B_{12} in the blood. The diagnosis of pernicious anemia is made by the Schilling test, which shows the failure of the gastrointestinal tract to absorb vitamin B_{12} unless intrinsic factor is given. Other, less common, causes of vitamin B_{12} deficiency include diseases of the small bowel (regional enteritis) and adherence to a strict vegetarian diet.

Treatment of pernicious anemia with monthly vitamin B_{12}

injections is all that is needed. Vitamin B$_{12}$ injections are of no value for any other illness or disease, however.

Marrow Failure. Anemia may develop if the factory (that is, the bone marrow) is unable to produce red cells at a proper rate. Normally, the marrow is able to increase its production six to eight times over normal to meet an increased demand, such as blood loss. Other disease processes, including chronic infection, long-standing kidney disease, cancer, or replacement of the marrow cavity with abnormal cells in leukemia or other malignant processes, can alter the ability of the marrow to make red cells, causing anemia.

Primary bone marrow failure or injury, called *aplastic anemia*, results in a depression of all the marrow elements, leading to a reduction in red blood cells, white blood cells, and platelets. The cause is often unknown, although at times exposure to certain drugs or chemicals can be implicated (such as chloramphenicol). This disorder is accompanied by anemia, bleeding tendencies, and repeated infections, often resulting in death. In some cases acute leukemia eventually develops.

Increased Destruction. Anemia may develop if the red blood cells are removed at an accelerated rate by the body. This condition, called *hemolysis*, occurs sometimes as an inherited disease. In some cases it may develop as an acquired abnormality by which the patient produces an antibody or protein that destroys his own red cells. This condition bears the designation autoimmune hemolytic anemia.

Genetic or inherited defects of the red cells may be of several types. There may be an abnormality in one of the proteins of the red cells called hemoglobin, which carries the oxygen and is made up of many building blocks called amino acids. If there is a substitution of one amino acid for another in the protein chain, the shape of the red cells changes, making them more rigid and vulnerable to destruction. This process of substitution of a different amino acid in the chain of the protein produces a disorder called a *hemoglobinopathy*. In sickle cell disease, an amino acid called valine is present instead of glutamine at the fifth part of the chain containing 143 amino acids. The mere replacement of one of 143 amino acids produces an abnormal hemoglobin called hemoglobin S. Red cells containing hemoglobin S may appear as sickle-shaped on the peripheral blood smear, hence the name *sickle cell anemia.*

Approximately 15 percent of all black persons in this country carry the abnormal hemoglobin S trait. Fortunately, these persons do not suffer from the sickle cell disease, because they receive two sets of genes (or hereditary traits), one from each parent. If one set of genes is normal, the person carries the abnormal genes from only one parent and is essentially free of disease except under circumstances of extreme oxygen deprivation. This occurred during World War II among military personnel during flights in nonpressurized airplane cabins. However, if two persons carrying the trait marry, as illustration 13 shows, the gene combinations of their children can be of three types. Some will merely "carry" the trait and be virtually symptom free. Another might receive the trait from both parents and suffer from sickle cell disease, and may have a decreased life expectancy as well as many painful episodes because of abnormal sickle cells. Other offspring may be perfectly normal. Approximately a half of one percent of all black persons in America have sickle cell disease, and currently, rapid screening tests are being employed to detect persons with the trait so that at least genetic counseling can be offered. Two persons with the trait should not marry each other, because each child they may have has a one in four chance of having sickle cell disease. The red cells of patients with this disease tend to sickle in certain blood vessels where the oxygen content is reduced. Sickled red cells tend to stagnate and block small blood vessels and produce blood clots in various body organs.

Another type of inherited disorder involves a reduction or absence of vital enzymes within the red cell itself. During its 120-day life span and its tortuous journeys in the body, the red cell is subject to many stresses and strains. A certain type of protein called an enzyme protects the membrane, or coat, of the red cell from injury and resulting disruption that would cause an early death of the cell. Certain drugs as well as infections can injure the red cell walls unless they are protected by enzymes. An inherited deficiency of an enzyme called glucose-6-phosphate dehydrogenase is present in many people, including whites from the Near East: Turkey, Iran, Greece, Israel, etc., as well as in some blacks. Some of these persons have a lifelong anemia, whereas others have an anemia only upon exposure to certain classes of drugs. This disorder is sex-linked, that is, it is carried by females, but usually affects only males.

Genetics of Sickle Cell Disease

If both parents are normal, a person inherits one normal gene (N) from each parent and can be represented as NN for this particular trait. If one parent has sickle cell disease, a person will inherit a sickle cell gene (S) as well as a normal gene (N) and have sickle cell trait (NS). Various possibilities are shown in the diagrams below:

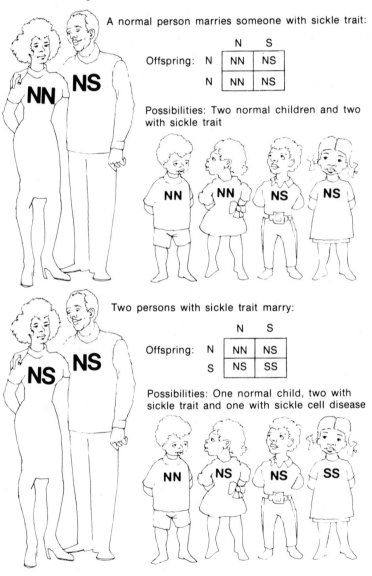

A normal person marries someone with sickle trait:

		N	S
Offspring:	N	NN	NS
	N	NN	NS

Possibilities: Two normal children and two with sickle trait

Two persons with sickle trait marry:

		N	S
Offspring:	N	NN	NS
	S	NS	SS

Possibilities: One normal child, two with sickle trait and one with sickle cell disease

Illustration 13

Another congenital or inherited defect in red cells is a condition called *hereditary spherocytosis*. These red cells are spherical rather than the normal biconcave disks, and are recognized as misshapen and removed prematurely by the spleen. Increased activity is required by the bone marrow to compensate for this loss. Many persons with this defect are not anemic unless subject to stress of an accompanying infection, such as a cold. A normal person has to replace 0.8 percent of the red cells every day, but a patient with this disturbance may be replacing 4 to 5 percent per day. During the stress of infection the marrow may markedly decrease production for several days. The normal person has virtually no detectable decrease in the number of red cells, whereas the patient with congenital spherocytosis may lose 25 to 50 percent of his red cells and become acutely ill.

Patients with the above types of congenital anemias are often jaundiced or yellow. Under normal circumstances, worn-out or destroyed red cells are disassembled in the body, the iron being recycled and reused, and the bilirubin, a yellow pigment, is excreted by the liver in the stools. Because of the increased destruction of red cells, a greater amount of bilirubin is formed, and this causes a yellowing of the skin or the eyes as the blood levels of bilirubin rise.

By unknown mechanisms, the bone marrow under normal circumstances maintains a relatively constant production of red cells. In our homes, a thermostat maintains the desired temperature. A similar control exists in the body to maintain a constant level of red blood cells. As we have discussed, anemia represents a decreased number of red cells. An overproduction of red blood cells may also occur, and this is called *polycythemia*. The causes of increased numbers of red cells are again multiple, and include a malignant or unchecked production of red cells analogous to leukemia, in which there is an increased number of malignant white cells. Patients with chronic lung disease who cannot adequately transfer oxygen into the blood also produce greater numbers of red cells to try to compensate for this defect.

The oxygen content of air is decreased in persons living and breathing at high altitudes, and accordingly their bone marrow normally makes greater numbers of red cells to carry the decreased amounts of available oxygen. Residents of Lima, Peru, and Denver, for example, have higher levels of red blood cells. Unusual causes of increased red cells include certain kidney diseases and some tumors of the uterus, liver, and cerebellum.

White Blood Cells

The white blood cells or leukocytes serve two main functions. Some white cells called neutrophils or polymorphs can surround, absorb, and digest bacteria. Other white cells called lymphocytes are involved in the manufacture of antibodies or proteins which protect the body from certain types of infectious agents. Lymphocytes become sensitized to foreign protein and are the cells that make antibodies during routine immunizations such as those for diphtheria, poliomyelitis, or tetanus. Following immunization, certain lymphocytes retain a "memory" against the foreign protein, often for a lifetime. The antibodies produced following certain viral illnesses, such as measles, protect us from repeated attacks.

The normal white blood cell count in a cubic millimeter of blood is between 5,000 and 10,000 cells. In bacterial infections, this count often is elevated, and in viral illnesses, it is generally normal or decreased. An example of how the white blood count helps the physician can be seen when a patient has a sore throat with some pus or exudate on his tonsils. There is no accurate and immediate way to determine whether this is caused by a bacterial infection, such as Streptococcus, or by one of many viral organisms. A streptococcal infection responds to penicillin and if untreated can occasionally cause rheumatic fever or certain types of kidney disorders. A viral illness does not respond to penicillin, and accordingly the drug should not be given. A culture of the throat would provide the answer in 48 hours. However, a patient often needs to be treated while the culture is pending, and if the white blood count is elevated and there are increased numbers of neutrophils, this suggests to the physician the presence of a bacterial or streptococcal infection. A normal white blood count and a normal number of neutrophils support a viral cause for the throat infection.

In viral illnesses, there is often an increase in the number of lymphocytes, and some of these are atypical in appearance and can be recognized from the blood smear. Infectious mononucleosis, a common disorder of young adults, is believed to be a viral illness, during which atypical lymphocytes are present, and together with certain other blood tests these cells confirm the diagnosis.

As with the red blood cells in anemia, there are disorders in which too few white cells are formed. Not only the number but the type of white cells is important. A person may have a normal white blood count but a relative increase in lymphocytes because of a decrease in neutrophils. This often occurs in a viral illness but may also represent a dangerous reaction to a drug because of selective injury to the neutrophil population.

In *leukemia*, there may be a striking increase in white cells, but only a primitive type is produced that cannot protect a patient against infections. Leukemia may represent a failure of the precursor or progenitor cells to mature toward useful white cells. The disease includes several different varieties of white cell disorders, reflecting a malignant change in the class of white cells that is involved.

Leukemias may be acute or chronic. Some of the latter types may be relatively harmless and may not shorten life, although generally these patients are more susceptible to certain types of infection. Acute leukemias, except in children, are usually rapidly fatal, with few patients surviving longer than one year in spite of intensive treatment. Death is generally due to overwhelming infections or catastrophic bleeding. There are promising developments in the treatment in childhood, with many patients living longer than three years and an increasing number of actual cures.

Platelets

Platelets serve a vital function. They form a basic mechanism for clotting along with proteins called *clotting factors* circulating in the blood. When we cut ourselves, after a variable period of bleeding, the wound coagulates or ceases to bleed. Coagulation or clotting requires the participation of platelets as well as clotting factors. A disrupted capillary or blood vessel is sealed by plugs of platelets, which adhere to the injured vessel wall and in the process release substances that enable clotting factors in the blood to form fibrin. Fibrin together with the plug of platelets seals the injured blood vessel and causes bleeding to stop.

If the number of platelets in the blood is reduced, bleeding tendencies may develop. If the level is quite low, serious bleeding from the gastrointestinal tract or nose and bruising of the skin may occur. If the level is only slightly reduced, symptoms may not be present. Bruising and actual bleeding are the two main manifestations of a decreased number of platelets. Platelets are also known as thrombocytes, and a decreased number of platelets is known as thrombocytopenia. Many different disorders can cause a reduction in the number of platelets in the blood. In children, acute infections, such as measles or other viral illnesses, are often accompanied by such a decrease. Generally this reduction is only temporary and no treatment is necessary.

In some persons, although the bone marrow seems to be producing adequate numbers of platelets, these platelets are destroyed in the blood by an antibody. This condition, called immune thrombocytopenia purpura, may respond to a cortisone-type of drug, or in some cases surgical removal of the spleen may be necessary. The spleen is a large lymph node in the abdomen that normally removes worn-out blood cells, and blood cells that it recognizes as abnormal because of differences in shape or because of antibody coating the surface of the cells.

Certain drugs can cause a reduction in the number of platelets because antibodies directed against the drug react with the platelet and destroy it in the process. Certain patients develop this sensitivity to quinine or quinidine and produce antibodies against these drugs. "Cocktail purpura" is a condition that may occur in patients who develop antibodies to quinine and experience bruising after they consume gin and tonic (which contains quinine).

A few susceptible persons have a temporary decrease in platelets following excessive consumption of alcohol. Persons who receive multiple blood transfusions with blood that has been stored in a blood bank rather than fresh blood also may have decreased platelets. The red cells survive in blood collected for transfusion for up to 21 days, whereas the platelets are no longer present after 24 to 48 hours. As with red blood cells and white blood cells, certain persons may have an abnormal increase in platelets in the blood.

Aspirin has a profound effect on the proper functioning of platelets. The ability of platelets to adhere to one another and form a plug can be interfered with by one aspirin tablet for up to several days after its ingestion. Aspirin can increase or aggravate a bruising tendency or even cause blood loss from the gastrointestinal tract, not only because of a direct irritation on the stomach wall but also by crippling the ability of platelets to function properly. This effect of aspirin on the platelet is sometimes used in an attempt to prevent abnormal clotting in blood vessels, the goal being to prevent strokes and heart attacks.

Bleeding Disorders

Bleeding disorders may be due to a decrease in the number of platelets or their capacity to function properly. An injury such as a hard blow to the arm may produce a bruise, which is caused by rupture of tiny blood vessels or capillaries and leakage of blood into the tissues. Women are particularly sensitive to bruising. Elderly persons also bruise easily because aging makes blood vessels more fragile.

A small number of patients have bleeding problems because the plasma proteins or clotting factors that are necessary in normal clotting are decreased or absent. The classic example is *hemophilia*, usually transmitted to males by their unaffected mothers. This genetic pattern is called sex-linked, since only males are victims while females are carriers of the gene or trait. Hemophilia has been known for more than 2,000 years and has affected certain branches of European royal families. However, there can be deficiencies of other serum proteins beside factor VIII, the antihemophilia factor, and most are not sex-linked, that is, they involve both males and females. Patients with diseases involving the liver may not be able to manufacture these various clotting factors and may be prone to bleeding disturbances.

Blood banking techniques now enable the factor VIII in blood to be separated and stored. Patients with hemophilia can periodically receive factor VIII concentrates to prevent major bleeding episodes and to maintain adequate levels of factor VIII in their blood, permitting a more normal life pattern. Home programs have been established where patients can administer factor VIII preparations to themselves. Plasma transfusions can be used to correct deficiencies of most of the other clotting factors in emergencies created by bleeding episodes.

Anticoagulants

Anticoagulants are administered to patients in order to prevent clotting in the body. In persons who have clots in their legs because of inflammation in their veins, or phlebitis, there is the risk that the clots will dislodge from their veins, travel to the lungs, and cause death by obstructing the flow of blood. "Blood thinners" (a commonly used but not very accurate term) or *anticoagulants* are given to prevent new clots from forming while the normal defense mechanisms of the body remove previously formed ones through lysis, or digestion. Patients who are bedridden for long periods of time, such as after surgery or a heart attack, can develop blood clots because of poor flow, or stasis of blood, in their legs. This problem can often be reduced by anticoagulants.

The usual anticoagulants work by interfering with the formation of the fibrin clot. There are two main types of anticoagulants: heparin, which is injected into a vein and which acts instantaneously, and coumarin derivatives, which are given by mouth but take two to three days to become effective. Heparin works by blocking the formation of fibrin; the coumarin drugs, such as Coumadin or Dicumarol, work by interfering with the production of the clotting factors in the liver which eventually participate in forming fibrin.

Blood Products and Blood Donations
Many patients require blood products because of illness. The benefits of modern-day surgery are largely due to the ability to replace blood lost during surgery by means of blood transfusions. Also, we can now furnish the patient with components of blood rather than whole blood. A patient with chronic anemia requires red blood cells and does not need whole blood, which contains plasma. In fact, the additional volume of whole blood can precipitate heart failure in such a recipient. The plasma can further be separated into platelets and clotting factors, such as factor VIII. The latter can be frozen and available to treat a hemophiliac patient. A blood donor may provide blood products to several patients. One may receive the prepared platelets, another the red cells, a third the factor VIII, and the remaining plasma may be used to prepare gamma globulin, the portion of blood containing antibodies.

Although the treatment of many diseases requires blood and its products, in this country there is a shortage of blood because many healthy people fail to participate in blood procurement programs, despite the vigorous efforts of the Red Cross. There is no reason why a healthy person who is not currently taking medications should not give blood several times a year. There is no substitute for blood.

Symptoms you should know about:

Weakness, pale skin, short-windedness, and palpitations are frequent symptoms of anemia, the commonest of blood disorders. Other important blood disorders may show up as **swollen glands** in the neck, armpits, or groin, or as **abnormal bleeding,** such as nosebleed, vomiting or coughing up blood, and passage of blood in urine or stools, or from the vagina. One special form of abnormal bleeding is **purpura,** or bleeding in the skin, which may look like tiny red dots or be large "black and blue" marks.

CANCER 12

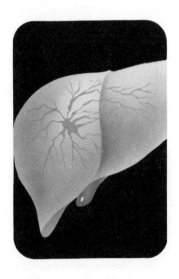

Cancer is among the most dreaded diseases of mankind. It accounts for a great loss of human life and resources each year, often taking its toll during our most productive years. It affects all age groups, and spares no race or economic class. The anguish of relatives and friends as they watch their loved one gradually deteriorate and succumb to cancer is immeasurable.

Cancer can occur in any organ of the body. It is almost always fatal if untreated. The outlook for long-term survival varies with the location and extent of the disease. In skin cancers, the chances for a cure are as high as 95 percent. Other types of cancers may be fatal in just a few months.

Despite millions of dollars spent at our best research centers and the efforts of many dedicated and able scientists, the mysteries of cancer—its causes and effective treatment— remain largely obscure. Our main goal—*prevention*—is not currently possible for most types of cancer. *Detection* is often too late for surgical or other cure, and *treatment* is often ineffective.

Yet some form of treatment exists for almost all kinds of cancer. The American Cancer Society estimates that 1,500,000 Americans who have been treated for cancer have now been free of their disease for at least five years. In 1978, 700,000 new cases of cancer were diagnosed.

What is Cancer?

Cancer represents an abnormality in the growth of some of the body's cells. Almost all human tissue undergoes some degree of cell replacement except for the brain and probably muscle. Some human tissues, such as the bone marrow and the cells lining the gastrointestinal tract, have a high cell turnover, but most human tissue is undergoing some growth and new cell formation to balance cell loss and death. Millions of cells are being replaced daily in various organs by a complex process called mitosis, whereby the nucleus and its DNA content double and the cell then divides into two daughter cells. If a large part of an organ such as the liver is removed experimentally, a burst of new cell activity and growth occurs until the organ has returned to its approximate former size. The cell growth does not continue beyond this point; once a critical mass is established in any given tissue or organ of the body, a state of equilibrium is reached and cell growth approximates cell loss.

In cancer tissue, groups of cells no longer remain under the normal control mechanisms of cell growth. Cancer cells continue to proliferate or multiply wildly, until the host, that is, the patient, is destroyed as the volume of cancer tissue reaches a certain size or damages a vital organ.

Cells of most human tissues perform distinct functions. As they mature, human cells develop differently in human organs so that a kidney cell looks different under a microscope from a heart muscle cell. In cancer tissue, the cells sometimes resemble the tissue of origin, but most often are more primitive or undifferentiated in appearance. Physicians called pathologists are trained to recognize cell patterns and differences by studying the appearance of resected tissue or biopsy material submitted by surgeons for analysis.

Thus two features of cancer tissue make it recognizable as malignant: 1. The cancer cells are usually more primitive in appearance, and no longer reflect the differentiation of tissue that occurs in order to perform specific functions. 2. The cancer cells are no longer under the control mechanism of orderly cellular growth; cancer tissue can grow and spread throughout the body, or metastasize, until the patient eventually succumbs.

Doctors often talk about tumors. Although strictly speaking tumor simply means a swelling, the term as ordinarily used refers to growth of tissues or cells. Tumors may be *benign* or *malignant*. Benign tumors do not grow endlessly and, therefore, do not endanger the host. A lipoma or fatty tumor is a common benign tumor. A malignant tumor is a cancerous tumor. In a sense, cancer is a biological mistake, for the cancerous tissue is parasitic (can exist only by deriving its nourishment from the host) yet by proliferating and destroying the host, it, too, dies.

Since millions of cells each day are undergoing complex growth processes ultimately leading to cell division, it is not surprising that something may go wrong and that a deranged or altered cell is produced.

Normally the lymphocytes in our blood and in certain tissues such as lymph nodes can recognize foreign tissue, for example viruses and other infectious organisms as well as transplanted tissue such as a kidney or heart transplant. Lymphocytes may also recognize altered host cells (potential cancer cells) as foreign tissue, and act to reject them. Potential cancer cells may be formed in all of us daily. These cells are then recognized as abnormal, or foreign, by our lymphocytes, and removed. Cancer may represent a breakdown of this normal internal surveillance system by unknown factors.

This conclusion is suggested by the high incidence of cancers that develop in persons born with deficiency of lymphoid tissue, who have defective or decreased numbers of lymphocytes in their body. More evidence comes from patients who receive organ transplants such as a kidney or heart, and whose lymphocytes would normally reject the foreign organs (unless from an identical twin or family member with the same tissue type). Drugs are given to prevent the lymphocytes from rejecting the organ. However, patients given these so-called immunosuppressant drugs have a much higher incidence of certain types of cancer. A cancer called reticulum cell sarcoma normally occurs in approximately 1 in 50,000 persons; but in 2,000 patients who had kidney transplants and who received immunosuppressant drugs, 12 reticulum cell sarcomas developed, or 300 times the expected incidence!

Predisposing Factors

The causes of most cancers are unknown. Over the years, many factors have been studied and some have been shown to be somehow related to certain types of human cancer. Radiation exposure, viral disease, racial influences, diet, chemicals, and occupational and other environmental factors have been implicated in certain types of tumors.

Radiation.   Radiation exposure is known to predispose to certain types of cancer. Many of the early workers with x-rays, who were improperly screened from high doses of radiation, eventually developed skin cancers. In the 1930s in this country, women working in a watch factory used radium paint to produce fluorescent numbers on watch dials; the technique involved wetting the paint brush with the tongue and dipping the brush into the paint, and many workers subsequently developed cancers of the head and neck. Persons exposed to atomic radiation at Hiroshima and Nagasaki have a higher incidence of thyroid cancer. Radiation used to treat acne in adolescents, and x-ray treatment of children for enlargement of the thymus gland, are now known to be associated with an increased incidence of thyroid and skin cancer. Persons in England with a certain form of arthritis of the spine were often greatly improved with x-ray treatment to the spine, but many later developed acute leukemia. Other examples of associations between radiation and an increased incidence of certain types of cancer could be cited. Diagnostic x-rays are no longer a threat in this area because of technical improvements in the machines that have greatly reduced the dosage of x-rays required for these studies.

Viruses.   For many years certain viruses have been known to cause cancer in animals. Some strains of mice have a high frequency of breast cancer and others have a low incidence. If newborn mice from a strain with a low incidence are fed milk from mice of the strain with a high incidence, they later develop breast cancers in abnormally large numbers. The factor in mice milk that causes breast cancer was shown to be a virus, thus demonstrating the passage of a tumor-causing (oncogenic) virus from the mother to her children. Viruses which cause many animal tumors may play a role in human cancer.

A herpes virus called the Epstein-Barr virus appears to have an association with a common African tumor called Burkitt's lymphoma, as well as tumors of the cervix and tumors of the nasopharynx. No definite tumor cause and effect relationship has yet been conclusively established in man.

Racial and Dietary.   The World Health Organization maintains statistical data on the incidence of various types of cancers. Some countries have a high incidence of certain cancers, others a low one.

The Chinese have a high incidence of cancer of the liver compared to the rate in this country and other western countries. Cancer of the breast is quite common in the Parsu women of India compared to other Indian women. The Japanese have a high incidence of cancer of the stomach and a low incidence of cancer of the colon. In this country, cancer of the stomach is decreasing in frequency and cancer of the colon has become the commonest malignant tumor.

Geographic differences in certain cancers disappear in migrant populations in which the cancer rate approaches those of the native population, suggesting the role of external factors in determining cancer rates. Japanese who migrated to Hawaii have a higher incidence of cancer of the colon compared to those residing in Japan, yet lower than other Americans. The Nisei, second and third generation Americans of Japanese origin, have an incidence of cancer of the colon similar to other Americans. The native African has a low incidence of colon cancer, and has a diet high in roughage and low in processed carbohydrates, which is associated with a relatively greater number of daily bowel movements. Some researchers have theorized that there may be a relationship between the amount of fiber or the number of bowel movements per day and cancer of the colon. Jewish men have a low incidence of cancer of the penis and Jewish women a low incidence of cancer of the cervix. It has been suggested that circumcision performed on all Jewish male children, which has a religious origin, may play a role in this decreased incidence.

Occupational. That occupational exposure could influence cancer development has been known since the 18th century, when Sir Percival Potts commented on the high frequency of cancer of the scrotum among chimney sweeps. Workers in the aniline dye industry have an increased risk of cancer of the bladder. Recently an increase in lung cancer has been reported among male factory workers exposed to chloromethyl methylether (CMME). Persons working in uranium mines have long been known to have a high incidence of lung cancer. Many years after the original exposure, tumors called mesotheliomas may develop in those who have inhaled asbestos fibers. A chemical commonly used in the plastics industry, polyvinyl chloride, has been associated with a high incidence of liver cancer.

Environmental. The role of environmental pollutants as potential carcinogens (capable of causing cancer after exposure) is currently under active investigation. The main sources of air pollution are exhaust fumes from motorized traffic and smoke from heating fuels and industrial wastes. Several authorities have speculated that as much as 80 percent of all cancer is environmental in origin, but a study by the California State Department of Public Health failed to find an increased incidence of lung cancer in residents of Los Angeles where photochemical air pollution levels are the highest in California. Cigarette smoking is definitely related to cancer of the lung, and the incidence increases with the number of packs smoked per day and the years of smoking. This led to the Surgeon General's issuing a warning to cigarette smokers and a law requiring that the label on all cigarette packages state that cigarette smoking is dangerous to health.

Recently, a high incidence of cancer of the vagina has been reported in young women whose mothers received, many years earlier, estrogen drugs, given early in pregnancy to prevent a threatened abortion or miscarriage.

There are many more examples of associations within various population groups of cancer and dietary, environmental, and occupational factors. How various carcinogens induce malignant transformation of cells is under intensive investigation.

The Common Cancers

After skin cancers, the three most common cancers are cancer of the colon (including the rectum), cancer of the lung, and breast cancer. (See illustration 14.) In recent years there has been some improvement in the results of treatment if surgical cure is not achieved on the original attempt. The available alternate forms of treatment if the disease is not cured by surgery include radiation therapy and drug therapy, called *chemotherapy*. Radiation and chemotherapy have little if any effect on survival in most forms of lung cancer, and only perhaps 30 percent of patients with disseminated colon cancer benefit from drug treatment.

Lung Cancer. Approximately seventy-five thousand people die annually in America of lung cancer. This disease was relatively uncommon at the turn of the century but has increased sharply, paralleling the rise of cigarette smoking in this country. Initially almost exclusively a disease of men, its

Cancer Statistics

Estimated Incidence of Cancer in 1979*

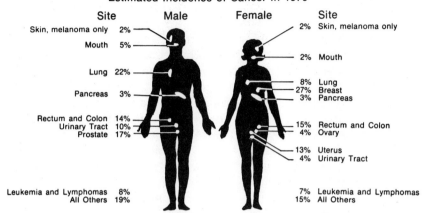

Estimated Cancer Deaths in 1979*

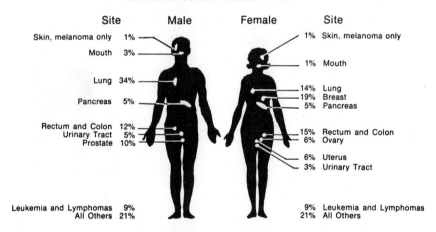

*Source: American Cancer Society, New York.

Illustration 14

frequency has been rising in women as they have taken up cigarette smoking.

Chest x-ray offers the best method for detecting lung cancer in asymptomatic persons. Often, even at this point, despite its having produced no symptoms, the cancer is beyond cure. The symptoms of lung cancer, such as a cough, sputum, or shortness of breath, are common in many cigarette smokers, so they are nonspecific. Hemoptysis, or coughing up of blood, deserves prompt evaluation including a chest x-ray and bronchoscopy, which is the passage of an instrument into the bronchial tubes to search for a tumor and collect samples of tissue for examination under the microscope for abnormal cells. Symptoms that may indicate lung cancer are often late signs.

Surgery is the treatment of choice to determine the nature of an abnormal mass or shadow on the chest x-ray if no other disease (such as tuberculosis) can be implicated. In cancer of the lung, only removal of the involved lobe of the lung offers a chance for cure. However, at the time of diagnosis or exploration of the chest by the surgeon, 65 to 80 percent of patients cannot undergo surgical resection because the disease is too widespread. The five-year survival for all persons with cancer of the lung is about 7 percent.

Prevention of lung cancer depends on a massive campaign of public education to stop smoking in established smokers and major efforts in our schools and our homes directed toward convincing children of the dangers of cigarette smoking. Perhaps a safe cigarette will be developed by the cigarette industry once the factors in cigarettes that induce cancer are clearly known. Efforts are under way to develop inexpensive screening of sputum by special stains (Papanicolaou technique) to detect suspicious cells in cigarette smokers. Currently, the yearly chest x-ray in smokers remains the only measure of value in early detection of cancer of the lung.

Cancer of the Breast.   Breast cancer is the major cause of cancer deaths in American women. Over 30,000 women die, and over 80,000 new cases of breast cancer develop yearly.

Cancer of the breast occurs more commonly in women who have a family history of cancer of the breast (mother or sister). Women who have had cancer of one breast are more likely to have a cancer in the remaining breast. In fact, one study showed that approximately 16 percent of women at the time of breast surgery have evidence of early, microscopic breast cancer in the other breast. There is no evidence that women who use birth control pills have any increase in the subsequent development of breast cancer.

Surgery is the only cure for this disease. Early detection, at a time when the breast mass is smallest, improves the overall results and survival. The method of surgery remains controversial. The radical mastectomy as popularized by the first professor of surgery at Johns Hopkins Hospital, William Halsted, remains a most commonly performed operation. This involves removal of the breast and underlying muscle tissue as well as a dissection and removal of axillary (armpit) tissue. A modified radical mastectomy, with preservation of some muscle tissue, has become more popular in recent years. A "superradical" operation, in which there is also removal of tissue beneath the breast bone, has also been attempted in an effort to improve overall results.

In Scotland, removal of the breast tissue (simple mastectomy) with preservation of underlying muscles, combined with postoperative radiation to the chest wall and axilla has gained considerable popularity as a method of treatment. The best 10-year results have occurred in series that have used the radical mastectomy. Early breast cancer—small tumors less than 2 centimeters in size or even smaller ones detected by breast x-ray examinations—has responded well to removal of the lump (lumpectomy) followed by radiation treatment to the breast, chest wall, and adjacent lymph node areas, thus preserving the breast and maintaining good cosmetic appearances. The results thus far for treatment of this type of breast cancer are most encouraging.

The complications of mastectomy include the great mental anguish that a woman experiences in losing a breast and, in a sense, what she may consider part of her womanhood. Some women experience swelling of the involved arm and may have some limitation in the use of the shoulder and arm. Physical therapy and exercise training can usually preserve full use of the involved arm. Specially fitted elastic appliances can be worn on the arm to prevent excessive swelling.

Breast cancers are notorious for their late recurrences. The presence of tumor spread to lymph nodes removed from under the arm at the time of the initial surgery indicates a high likelihood of eventual spread of the disease. The absence of tumor in the lymph nodes augurs a favorable outcome. Physicians often talk about 5-year survivals following cancer surgery as indicative of a good chance for permanent cure. This is not so for breast cancers. There have been recurrences of breast cancer as long as 20 years after the original surgery. Unlike the case in some lung cancers and in many cases of colon cancer, effective treatment is available for recurrent or metastatic breast cancer. Radiation, drugs, hormones, and further surgery to remove the ovaries or adrenal glands are available and effective in some patients. Women in whom cancer recurs who are still menstruating should have their ovaries removed, since this helps about one-third of patients. Later, patients who have shown improvement after removal of the ovaries may benefit from removal of the adrenal glands. Other persons benefit from various cancer drugs, some given in combination. Approximately 50 to 60 percent of persons improve with these drugs, occasionally for several years. Women who are postmenopausal may benefit from female hormones, called estrogens, male hormones, called androgens, or a new class of drugs called antiestrogens. The decision as to which type of treatment—whether additional surgery (removal of ovaries or adrenal glands), the use of various hormones, or chemotherapy—depends on information obtained by a test on the original breast cancer tissue, called the estrogen binding receptor test.

It is estimated that 90 percent of women who develop cancer of the breast discover their own breast lump and seek medical attention. Unfortunately, many women delay reporting a lump or breast mass for several weeks or months, hoping it will disappear. This delay undoubtedly decreases the chance for cure for some of them. The need for widespread instruction in self-examination of the breasts and the regular performance of this simple measure cannot be overstressed. Any suspicious breast mass should be evaluated by a physician.

Special x-rays of the breast called *mammograms* are often helpful in diagnosing breast cancer, as are other techniques such as xerography and thermography. The value of mass screening of a suitable age group (over the age of 50), has demonstrated the ability to see early cancers that are not yet large enough to be felt. Mammography is indicated in helping to evaluate any single mass in the breast or in lumpy or cystic breasts, in women who have already had one breast cancer, or in women who have a family history of breast cancer. The cost of screening large population groups by mammography in terms of the yield of abnormal results has not made this procedure as widespread as it deserves to be. All suspicious breast lumps should be biopsied (removed by a surgeon) in a hospital and the nature of the disease determined by the pathologist. If the tumor is benign, no further treatment is usually necessary; if malignant, appropriate surgery is performed.

Cancer of the Colon. Early detection of this cancer increases the survival rate. If the tumor is confined to the mucous membrane or inner lining of the bowel, and has not penetrated through the outer wall, chances for surgical cure remain relatively good. Mass screening of stool samples using Hemoccult cards can detect the presence of trace amounts of blood and is an effective method to identify patients who need further evaluation of the large bowel. Periodic evaluation of the lower bowel can be performed by a procedure called proctosigmoidoscopy, which involves passage of an instrument into the anal opening and through the rectum and lowermost colon as far as possible. Many colon cancers lie within the range of this instrument. A newer, flexible tube called a colonoscope is now available which allows visualization of most of the colon above the 25-centimeter (10 inch) range of the proctosigmoidoscope.

All rectal bleeding in persons over the age of 30 should be evaluated by proctosigmoidoscopy. If no cause is detected, a barium enema x-ray can be done to determine possible causes of bleeding. Although cancer of the colon has to be considered, hemorrhoids, fissures, polyps (which are most often benign tumors) and diverticuli are other possible causes.

If the cancer is located in the last portion of the colon, the rectum, surgery involves closure of the anal opening and establishing a new opening in part of the colon brought out through the abdominal wall—a procedure called a colostomy.

Treatment of widespread cancer of the colon or recurrent disease is mostly by means of certain drugs, especially 5-fluorouracil. Some newer drugs currently being used also appear promising.

Treatment

Some progress in cancer treatment with powerful drugs has occurred during the last 15 years. Chemotherapy employing combinations of various drugs has made substantial gains in improving survival in cancer of the ovary, bladder, small cell cancer of the lungs, uterine cancer, head and neck malignancies, lymph node cancers called lymphomas, and, as mentioned previously, breast cancer. It is possible to cure several types of cancer by the use of chemicals, often combined with radiation or surgery. Cures have been achieved in certain types of testicular cancer, Burkitt's lymphoma, retinoblastoma, neuroblastoma, rhabdomyosarcoma, Wilms' tumor, choriocarcinoma, childhood leukemia, and Hodgkin's disease.

The majority of these cancers are uncommon. Childhood leukemia accounts for nearly half of the deaths due to cancer in children between the ages of three and fifteen years. Current treatment allows for survival for longer than five years—compared to a survival of just a few months ten to fifteen years ago—and cure in up to 50 percent of these cases.

The treatment of Hodgkin's disease, a cancer of the lymph nodes, has also been significantly improved by new techniques of x-ray therapy and, in advanced cases, the use of several drugs simultaneously. A complete remission can be obtained in 80 percent of cases, and many of these patients can achieve further remissions after relapse. An increasing, percentage of Hodgkin's disease victims can be completely cured.

A currently promising avenue of research is in the area of immunotherapy. The cancer patient's lymphocytes can, like normal lymphocytes, kill cancer cells. Stimulation of this system has proved beneficial in some persons with melanoma, a malignancy arising in certain cells of the skin. Further knowledge may help us apply immunotherapy more widely in treating cancer.

Symptoms you should know about:

The symptoms of cancer may be either constitutional (involving the whole body) or referable to the location of the malignant process. Depression, poor appetite, weight loss, weakness, and fever are examples of the former sort. Clues to specific forms of cancer are **bleeding** from any part of the body, abnormal **swelling of lymph nodes** or of abdominal organs, or a **lump** in the breast.

BRAIN AND PERIPHERAL NERVES

13

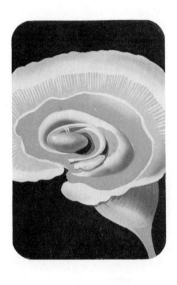

Headache

A physician was telling about a brilliant diagnosis he had made. A young married nurse came to him because of severe headaches she had been having for many weeks. After a few minutes of questioning her, he made the diagnosis of a brain tumor, which was subsequently confirmed and successfully treated. His colleague said that was very interesting and added that he'd done the same thing on two or three occasions himself. His doctor friend grinned triumphantly, as though he'd expected him to say that, then explained that he'd diagnosed the brain tumor *in the patient's husband!* He had quickly determined that the nurse's headaches were caused by anxiety, and that she was worried about her husband's bizarre behavior; the pattern of this behavior suggested brain irritation from the presence of a mass.

This true story illustrates some important medical facts about headache. First, an organically sound person, the nurse, suffered from severe headache, although the most careful physical examination and exhaustive medical testing would have failed to find anything wrong with her. And second, her husband, with a large tumor pressing on his brain, had no headache at all. Let us consider some anatomy to see how such paradoxical things can be explained.

251

Pain is a specific sensation that we experience when certain areas of our brain are stimulated by impulses brought to those areas by nerve fibers. Although we feel pain in a fingertip when we strike it with a hammer, the pain sensation really depends upon the pain center in the brain receiving the message from the hurt fingertip. If the delivery of the message is blocked by cutting the nerve fibers involved or by "blocking" the nerves with an anesthetic, we won't feel pain even though we mash the finger with a hammer. Normally nerve endings in the skin and underlying tissues are stimulated by injury, and these nerves conduct an impulse to the spinal cord, and up the cord to the thalamus, a structure deep inside the brain, and then to the cortex, or outer layer of the brain. When it reaches the cortex we then experience pain in the area where those nerve endings are situated, as shown in illustration 15.

The skull and the brain tissue itself do not have nerve endings that lead to the thalamus and pain centers in the cortex, so they can be struck or even cut through without pain. Some brain operations are done with the patient under a local anesthetic, that is, the skin and underlying tissues are rendered pain-free by injection of a drug to temporarily block the nerves in the area of the injection. Then the surgeon can saw through the skull and cut through the brain tissue and the patient will not feel a thing.

This is why a brain tumor can squeeze the brain considerably and still not cause pain. Then why do some brain tumors or other disease inside the skull cause headaches? There are pain-sensitive structures inside the skull, even though the brain itself is not one of these; the arteries, some veins, part of the covering of the brain at the base, and several cranial nerves can all set up nerve impulses that cause pain. Traction, displacement, and inflammation of these sensitive tissues can be responsible for headache. So the location of the disease process inside the skull determines whether the patient feels pain in his head.

Most headaches arise in tissues located outside the skull. All the tissues of the head and face outside the skull are pain-sensitive. These include the skin, all the many blood vessels, the lining of the sinuses, and muscle and fascia. This last, fascia, is a layer of loose connective, or fibrous, tissue, with variable amounts of fat, which is present under the skin. The fascia is richly supplied with nerves and blood vessels. It differs in thickness, being thin over the forehead and thick

The Pain Pathway

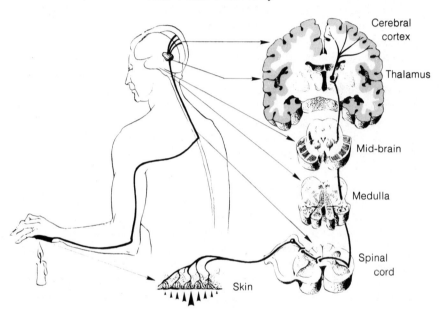

Illustration 15

and tough over the scalp. Strong muscles lie over the bones of the skull and are an important source of headache. When these muscles contract tightly, nerve endings are stimulated and headache results.

Very few adults have not had at least one headache in their lives, and many persons have had innumerable headaches. Most headaches disappear spontaneously or respond to simple pain medication, such as aspirin. The enormous quantities of aspirin used for headaches, and the wide variety of patent medicines sold for this purpose, testify to the vast numbers of headaches experienced in the world today.

The most common cause of headache is chronic anxiety and emotional tension. Under these circumstances many persons react with sustained contraction of the scalp muscles and associated constriction of the many arteries in these muscles. Vascular headaches, including migraine, are the next most common. Then, in order of frequency, come headaches associated with dehydration and fever, and then those due to sinus and nose and eye diseases. Relatively rare but most important to the victim are the headaches from brain tumors and abscesses, meningitis, aneurysms at the base of the brain, and similar serious but unusual diseases.

Not all tense people have headaches, and why some do is not known. All people with headaches due to emotional tension do not feel tense. It is thought then that the tension is converted into headache rather than the unpleasant emotional expression that another person may feel.

Chronic anxiety may cause several sorts of head discomfort. One common result of longstanding tenseness is a feeling of constriction, which many sufferers insist is a different sensation from pain, located in a circle around the head, in what doctors call a "hat-band" distribution. Another common complaint of tense persons is a vague discomfort that cannot be localized within the head, that is, the person can't say whether it is on the left or right side or front or back.

The classical *tension headache* often begins in the back of the head or neck, then extends over the top to the forehead, so that it finally involves the entire head. Frequently, the headache develops in the frontal area only. It is often described as a constant pain. As the scalp muscles and fascia tighten, the skin of the scalp becomes tender, and where the muscle tension is very high in small areas, painful lumps may even appear on the scalp. Aspirin and similar simple pain medications are usually effective during the first few hours of this sort of headache, but once the scalp muscle tension becomes established, the spastic muscle may continue to cause pain for days at a time.

Migraine headaches have many causes, and many different circumstances may bring them on in different persons. Emotional upsets, the menstrual period, bright lights, loud noises, eating certain foods, etc., all may precipitate a migraine in a susceptible person. Frequently, no cause can be found.

A typical migraine attack may begin with an "aura," that is a warning that the headache is about to come. This can consist of visual disturbances, especially bright flashes of light or blind spots in half the field of vision or a vague uneasiness or a numbness of half the body or just a small part. The aura is caused by a constriction in the blood vessels in one half of the head. When the eye or the brain is predominantly involved, the symptoms as mentioned above may be very frightening. Difficulty in speaking or paralysis may even occur in rare cases. Fortunately, the aura is always brief, usually just a few minutes, and the person always recovers completely. Many times there is no aura at all, and occasionally the migraine attack stops after the aura without an ensuing headache.

The migraine headache usually involves one side of the head (hemicrania). Many persons experience it more often on one side or the other, and in many it occurs in either side with equal frequency. The pain itself is a very unpleasant throbbing, with severe pain occurring every time the heart beats. This is so because distension, stretching of the blood vessels of the scalp (vasodilatation), activates pain fibers in the wall of the artery, producing the headache. Nausea and vomiting often occur, and the headache may disappear after vomiting. More usually the throbbing pain lasts for several hours and is gradually replaced by a more constant pain over the entire head as a tension headache replaces the vascular headache.

Some sufferers can abort a migraine attack by rebreathing, that is, breathing into a paper bag and inhaling the already used air, which has a high carbon dioxide content. This trick is effective only during the aura, and if used during the headache phase may make it worse. Ergotamine-type medication (for example, Cafergot) may be spectacularly effective in a migraine attack if taken early. Aspirin, sedatives, and tranquilizers are often helpful, and rest in a quiet, dark room is usually effective. Methysergide (Sansert) is a drug successful in preventing migraine (although of no help once the attack has begun) but may cause serious side effects.

Migraine tends to run in families. It is more common in women, especially in adolescence and around the menopause. Such headaches generally disappear after the menopause.

Other sorts of vascular headaches are common in males, are of briefer duration, and may come on during sleep or in clusters, that is, frequently for a few days or weeks, and then none at all for long periods of time.

The doctor can often make the diagnosis of the sort of headache a person has fairly easily by taking the history of the headache and performing a thorough physical examination. Sometimes the cause is not obvious and further tests may be required to find (or better yet, to rule out) one of the serious but rare causes. Skull x-rays, brain waves (electroencephalograms), and radioisotope brain scans are commonly used. Arteriography, which is discussed in the section on cerebrovascular diseases, allows detailed study of the blood vessels of the brain. Recently, a new X-ray procedure (computerized axial tomography) allows doctors to examine the brain with greater detail than by all previous techniques. Study of cerebrospinal fluid obtained by lumbar puncture often yields valuable information.

Dizziness

All of us have experienced the feeling of dizziness or lightheadedness. The sensation reflects the input of sensory areas in our body, including the inner ear, into the balance center located in the hind brain or medulla. There are important connections to other areas of the brain, including the midbrain and cerebellum, as well as to the cortex.

Vertigo is a term used to describe a form of dizziness associated with a spinning or moving sensation either of the head or of objects within the environment such as the ceiling or floor. Children playing blindman's bluff, a game in which they are spun round and round and then abruptly stopped, are aware of this sensation. Lightheadedness, a floating sensation of the head, is another term used to describe mild dizziness. Motion sickness (seasickness, car sickness, etc.) are special forms of dizziness initiated by various forms of travel.

Any condition that interferes with blood flow to the brain can be associated with lightheadedness or dizziness. An extreme example would be cessation of the heartbeat; dizziness occurs within several seconds and precedes unconsciousness. A very common experience is the dizziness due to a rapid change in position, such as from a lying to a standing position. This is called postural dizziness.

Blood carries oxygen for the functioning and survival of brain cells. The flow of blood to the brain is uphill against the force of gravity, requiring the pumping action of the heart. When we assume the upright position after lying or sitting, blood tends to be trapped in our legs and the lower portions of the body. This pooling of blood temporarily diminishes the volume returning to the heart and would ordinarily decrease the amount to be pumped to the brain. However, several compensatory mechanisms occur rapidly. The blood vessels in our legs tend to constrict, narrowing their diameter and thereby their capacity to store large amounts of blood which would otherwise be unavailable for the heart to pump to the brain. Our heart rate also increases to maintain effective circulation to our vital organs. Dizziness can occur if we rapidly stand and there is a delay of several seconds in the reflex narrowing of blood vessels in the legs. This commonly occurs in otherwise healthy persons. It may be noted especially after a night's sleep when we are still groggy and stand quickly to answer a phone or to go to the bathroom. Bending over, for example, working in a garden, especially during a hot day, might cause transient dizziness when one stands up.

Elderly patients are more likely to experience postural dizziness. Aging is associated with thickening and hardening (arteriosclerosis) of blood vessels and narrowing of the arteries. A narrowed blood vessel can deliver less blood to vital areas of the brain even under normal circumstances. Therefore, rapid changes of position, by momentarily trapping blood in the legs, produces a critical reduction of blood flow to the brain and may lead to either dizziness or actual fainting.

Postural dizziness is not a serious problem in the average person. It can be readily diagnosed because it occurs with changes in position so that other potentially serious causes of dizziness can be excluded. Persons who experience this dizziness are encouraged to change position more slowly so that the normal adaptive mechanisms can be effective.

Older people can also have postural dizziness because of the additional effect of narrowed cerebral blood vessels. Sudden movement of the head up or down or side to side can cause kinking of blood vessels located in the neck and temporarily decrease blood flow to areas of the brain. The result is reduced oxygen delivery to brain cells, causing dizziness or even fainting.

Hyperventilation. One of the commonest forms of dizziness is due to hyperventilation. We all breathe, yet we are unaware on a minute-to-minute basis of the outward and inward movements of the chest wall as the lungs are inflated and deflated and gas exchange occurs.

Normally, we breathe 8 to 12 times per minute. Oxygen is transferred from our lungs into our blood, and carbon dioxide, a waste product of body metabolism, is excreted. If we breathe more rapidly, say, 15 or 20 times per minute, or more deeply, as in a sigh, we are overbreathing or hyperventilating; in the process, we blow off or excrete excess amounts of carbon dioxide. Carbon dioxide is an acid, and its deficit changes the normal blood acid concentration, producing a feeling of lightheadedness or dizziness.

The feeling of lightheadedness is real and is worrisome, especially if a relative or friend has had a stroke or heart attack, because of fear of a similar event and impending doom. The resulting anxiety initiates further hyperventilation, making the dizziness worse. At this point, numbness and tingling of the hands, fingertips, or lips may be present; the chest muscles are overworked and become sore; adrenalin is released into the blood, producing sweating and a rapid heart-rate or palpitations; a fullness in the lower chest develops because of distension of the stomach with swallowed air; belching is often present; and the person may actually faint. At this point, many patients are rushed to an emergency room by worried relatives.

The sequence of events cited above can be induced in all normal persons who are instructed to hyperventilate. Hyperventilation occurs most commonly in young people who are mildly depressed, anxious, or unhappy with their roles. It tends to occur during periods of inactivity, such as lying in bed or watching television, rather than when we are busily engaged in our usual chores or activities. During such periods, we often rehash the day's activities as well as past events that may not have turned out as we expected; we think about our jobs and work responsibilities. We may love our husbands or wives and children but find the role of parent or breadwinner boring or frustrating. Many ambivalent feelings are exposed, and unconsciously, we begin to hyperventilate. Smokers are affected by hyperventilation and become concerned about their heart and lungs during the overbreathing and associated chest wall fullness.

Physicians usually recognize the dizziness caused by hyperventilation. Often, as the patient discusses his symptoms, he is observed to be hyperventilating and taking periodic deep, sighing breaths. This reaction can be abolished by placing a bag over the mouth and nose and rebreathing the carbon dioxide that is being blown off during overbreathing. The physician can often reassure the patient by showing him that all the symptoms associated with hyperventilation will occur if he voluntarily overbreathes. Many patients describe the need to overbreathe as the sequence evolves, and once told that this causes the problem, can be taught to refrain from rapid and deep breathing. Nervous and anxious patients are often helped by a trial of tranquilizers, but most patients require no treatment once the cause of their lightheadedness is explained and reproduced.

Inner Ear Problems. Dizziness or vertigo may occur because of disorders in the inner ear balance centers or labyrinths. This condition may accompany a general infection in the upper respiratory area—nose, sinuses, and ears—as occurs during a cold, or may persist after the clearing of all the other symptoms of a head cold; sometimes, the dizziness is due to nonspecific causes of inflammation in the ear producing an acute or chronic labyrinthitis.

Persons who have an acute attack of vertigo associated with a cold or viral illness generally improve with treatment of the inflammation by decongestants and antihistamines. At times, the dizziness is so disabling that the person is unable to stand because of loss of balance. Any slight motion of the head activates the inflamed labyrinth, causing a severe spinning sensation, and the patient may stagger and fall.

A special form of dizziness due to disturbance in the inner ear is known as Ménierè's disease. This condition is associated with a progressive hearing loss along with a ringing sensation in the ears, as well as vertigo.

Many other disorders, such as severe cases of anemia, may be associated with dizziness. Brain tumors are an uncommon cause of dizziness and are usually associated with the appearance of other neurological deficits or symptoms.

When the physician is asked to evaluate the problem of dizziness, he must take a careful history, including a description of the dizziness, the provoking factors, and associated symptoms. After performing a careful examination, he is generally able to pinpoint the problem and recommend corrective measures.

Epilepsy

Epilepsy describes a syndrome, or group of symptoms, with some combination of loss of consciousness, disturbances of sensation or altered feeling of parts of the body, and convulsions, which are jerky or shaking movements of the entire body or parts of it. The terms epilepsy, seizures, fits, and convulsions are synonymous.

The condition is described in the writings of Hippocrates of 2500 years ago and is derived from the Greek word meaning "taking hold of." In past centuries, people who had epilepsy were thought to be possessed by evil forces or to have special mystical powers. They were either exalted or exiled and persecuted.

Although epilepsy can occur at any age, it usually begins before the age of 20. Seizures may occur only once in the life of an individual or many times in a single day. A seizure is believed to occur when a region of the brain (a group of brain cells called neurons) periodically undergoes excessive and disorderly activity.

The causes of epilepsy are numerous, and seizures may develop from primary disturbances of the brain with the seizure as the sole manifestation of brain dysfunction, or with other neurological signs and symptoms. Seizures also are seen with other disease processes that can affect brain function. The list of such conditions is quite long and includes advanced kidney disease or uremia, endstage liver disease, metabolic disturbances such as abnormal blood calcium levels, a low blood sugar such as with insulin overdose, or uncommon tumors, low levels of oxygen in the blood as with carbon monoxide poison or in chronic lung disease, metastatic tumors, withdrawal from excess alcohol consumption, and high fever in children (febrile convulsions).

Seizures Associated with Brain Diseases. Almost any process that damages brain tissue can cause epilepsy by altering the seizure threshold of a particular area of the brain. Injury, various infections and inflammatory processes, certain birth defects, cerebrovascular diseases, degenerative brain disease, and tumors of the brain may all cause epilepsy.

Serious head trauma, usually not minor concussions, may be followed by epilepsy days to months after the event. Generally, the seizure develops between six months and two years after the injury.

Approximately 50 percent of patients with brain tumors develop seizures, and in 10 percent it is the first sign of a brain tumor. Seizures also follow cerebrovascular disease including strokes and hemorrhage into the brain. Infections of the brain, including meningitis, encephalitis, and brain abscess as well as neurosyphilis, may be followed by epilepsy.

Despite the numerous disorders that can cause brain damage, leaving an area of brain tissue vulnerable to seizure activity, often no precipitating event can be identified. In such cases, the person is said to have idiopathic epilepsy. Seizures are usually divided into several categories, including grand mal (major epilepsy), petit mal (minor epilepsy), and psychomotor epilepsy, based upon differences in the symptoms and evolution of the seizure event.

Grand Mal Epilepsy. Grand mal epilepsy is the commonest type of seizure disorder. Often the person can feel a seizure developing because of certain sensations called an aura which generally precede the seizure or convulsions. The aura may be a tingling sensation or numbness of part of the body or a peculiar taste. A loss of consciousness occurs, and the victim falls to the ground as the convulsion begins with a violent tightening or spasm of all the muscles of the body. The eyes roll to one side, the teeth are clenched, often with blood and saliva staining the lips. Breathing ceases and the skin becomes blue. After a few seconds, the muscle tightness gives way to a rhythmic jerky movement of the extremities and breathing is restored. Gradually, the abnormal movements cease and the patient breathes normally, sweating and in deep coma, unresponsive to painful stimuli, often lying in a pool of urine due to incontinence. The patient gradually awakens but remains confused and drowsy for hours and has no recollection of the seizure except perhaps for the strange feeling or aura that preceded the convulsion. Often he awakens in a hospital aware of a tremendous aching due to the violent contractions of his muscles, with a headache and often other injuries sustained in his fall, including fractures or lacerations.

Repeated convulsions of this type over a period of hours

with no regaining of consciousness are known as status epilepsy, and they require major medical efforts to stop them.

Petit Mal.   Petit mal seizures are seen almost exclusively in children and adolescents. Periods of unconsciousness occur frequently, as often as several hundred times a day. Unlike grand mal seizures, in petit mal epilepsy the person does not fall down and has no warning or aura of a seizure. The attacks are so brief that they often go undetected. Complex activities such as walking or riding a bicycle may continue during the seizure. The victim may stop speaking for several seconds or fail to respond to a question and then proceed, unaware of his lapse of consciousness.

This type of seizure pattern may evolve into grand mal seizures as the patient grows older. Frequent episodes of petit mal can seriously interfere with learning and school performance.

Psychomotor Epilepsy.   This type of seizure is felt to originate from a part of the brain called the temporal lobe and is sometimes called temporal lobe epilepsy. These seizures last seconds to several minutes and are often preceded by an aura, consisting of a past dream or visual experience or even a peculiar smell. Convulsions usually do not occur, but bizarre movements of the lips or tongue such as chewing or smacking of the lips may be present. The person is able to perform complex activities such as dressing or driving a car during the seizure but when questioned or given a command is unable to respond. Eventually, as many as two-thirds of these patients develop generalized convulsions.

Diagnosis and Treatment.   When epilepsy develops in any patient, diagnostic efforts are begun to determine whether the expression of brain dysfunction is due to other disease processes, some of which have already been cited, or whether primary brain disease is present. Seizures are identified from a recording of the electrical activity of brain cells, called an electroencephalogram or E.E.G. Tiny electrodes are placed along the scalp and record the rhythmic electrical activity from both sides of the brain surface. The usual pattern of 8 to 10 per second alpha waves may be replaced by abnormal waves which can be slower and of a different amplitude than normal. In petit mal epilepsy, a typical abnormality develops consisting of a spike and wave pattern at a rate of 3 per second that abruptly stops at the end of the seizure.

Other diagnostic steps include studies of the blood supply

of the brain, called angiography (discussed in the section on strokes), brain scans using radioactive isotopes that concentrate in an abnormal fashion in diseased areas of the brain such as a blood clot or brain tumor, and a spinal tap or lumbar puncture, which measures the spinal fluid pressure as well as allowing for analysis of the fluid bathing the brain and spinal cord for various chemical determinations. A neurologist, who is a specialist in brain diseases, often aids in the diagnostic evaluation as well as in the management of the patient.

Seizures are usually controlled or reduced in frequency by several types of medications called anticonvulsants. In many patients, more than one drug is necessary to control epilepsy, and each case requires specific doses and combinations of drugs for optimal results. Usually a class of drugs called hydantoins, which include diphenylhydantoin (Dilantin) is used alone or with a barbiturate such as phenobarbital. A witness to a seizure can best help the victim by trying to keep him from injuring himself by padding him with cushions or a coat and by removal of dangerous objects from the vicinity. A common but harmful maneuver is to try to prevent the patient "from swallowing his tongue," by putting objects between his teeth. This damages the teeth and mouth, and insertion of fingers may result in bad lacerations to the good Samaritan.

Parkinson's Disease

Paralysis agitans or Parkinson's disease is named after James Parkinson, who described the clinical findings of the disease in 1817. This illness is due to a dysfunction in an area of the brain called the basal ganglia and produces the characteristic disorders of movements. The main features include tremor, generalized stiffness or rigidity leading to difficulty in walking and a slowness in all voluntary actions, and a marked decrease in natural expression and movement.

The disease affects men more often than women and generally develops in middle aged or elderly people. The disease tends to have a gradual onset and progresses slowly. In the majority of cases, no underlying cause can be identified, and there is no predictable relationship to trauma, arteriosclerosis, or other brain disease. It has followed brain infections, and a considerable number of cases developed following the epidemic of influenza in World War I, postencephalitic Parkinsonism.

Recently, a chemical important in the transmission of impulses between nerve tissues has been found markedly diminished in the basal ganglia, and this abnormality provides the rationale for effective treatment described below.

In a typical case, an elderly patient is brought to the doctor by a member of his family because of "general deterioration." The patient usually has been having difficulty getting about and may have fallen. He has the "shakes," his speech is at times difficult to comprehend, and saliva drools from the sides of his mouth. On examination, the elderly gentleman sits motionless, with an expressionless or masklike face. He has a coarse tremor of his hands which tends to disappear on purposeful movement. The tremors occur at four to six times a second. Especially noteworthy is a "pill rolling" motion of the thumb and index finger. The voice is shrill, with a delay in beginning a sentence, followed by rapid speaking in a monotone. The patient performs all voluntary movements slowly and stiffly. When asked to get up and walk, he rises slowly, his head bent forward, his back bowed, and his arms held away from his body with elbows bent. His steps are short and hurried, almost as if he were running. The diagnosis of Parkinson's disease is easily made on the basis of this constellation of signs.

The treatment of Parkinson's disease has been greatly improved over the past decade with the drug Levodopa (L-Dopa), which can penetrate the brain substance and replenish the dopamine content of the brain. Mild disease of recent onset is more apt to respond than severe, longstanding disease. While all symptoms tend to improve, rigidity and slowness of voluntary movement responds more than does the tremor. The drug has to be given under close medical supervision, with the dose increased gradually to the desired level without producing potentially serious side effects. Nausea and vomiting may develop during the initial phases of treatment.

Patients with Parkinson's disease are usually elderly, often with impaired memory and judgment. Their illness tends to cause social isolation, and they require psychological support as well as physical and occupational therapy.

Multiple Sclerosis

Multiple sclerosis or disseminated sclerosis is a common crippling disorder of the central nervous system (brain and spinal cord). It usually develops in persons between the second and fourth decades, affects both sexes equally, is more common in temperate climates, especially northern Europe, and afflicts the white races more than others.

The disorder is characterized by widespread or multiple areas of degeneration of the white matter of the brain (myelin) and spinal cord as opposed to the gray matter. This loss of myelin (demyelinization) followed by scarring, proceeds in different stages in various areas of the central nervous system. The particular symptoms an individual may experience depend on the particular area of the brain or spinal cord that is involved and the function of that tissue.

One feature of this illness is the tendency for it to have periods of remission (improvement of symptoms) followed by relapses (recurrences of previous symptoms as well as additional ones). Generally, the disease follows a prolonged course of many years. Initial complaints may be limited because of focal involvement, but gradually the symptoms become more generalized and disabling as the disease becomes progressively more disseminated.

The cause of multiple sclerosis is unknown. Recently, a viral cause has been proposed but not proved. The disease bears a striking resemblance to an illness in sheep called scrapie. This progressive neurological disease in sheep is caused by a virus, called a slow virus because it takes a long time from infection with the organism until manifestations of the disease develop. Brain tissue from a patient with multiple sclerosis can produce scrapie in sheep. A primitive tribe in New Guinea has a high incidence of a progressive neurological disease similar to multiple sclerosis, which spares the young and affects only the adults. In the past these people practiced cannibalism and often ate the brains of their enemies, suggesting incidental ingestion of a slow virus as the eventual cause of their disease.

The symptoms accompanying multiple sclerosis can be quite variable, since they depend on the areas of the central nervous system involved. The initial complaints usually consist of some combination of visual symptoms, such as loss of vision or double vision; intermittent weakness or loss of control of the limbs, usually but not invariably both legs, making walking difficult; sensory disturbances, such as numbness of a limb(s) or of a side of the face. Often initial manifestations include speech disturbances, tremors, dizziness, or even tic douloureux (described later).

After a period of time, most often many years, the disease

produces widespread scarring in many areas of the brain and spinal cord, leading to major neurological symptoms and handicaps. The patient may be bedridden and unable to walk because of paralysis of the limbs. Vision, speech, swallowing, sensation, mood or affect, movement coordination, and performance of complex acts may all be disturbed. Bladder and bowel functions are also commonly impaired late in the course of the illness.

The diagnosis of early multiple sclerosis may often be difficult, especially when only a single complaint such as dizziness is present. At the other extreme, in a patient seen with multiple areas of involvement, especially with periods of remission, diagnosis is usually easy. Finding of a high gamma globulin level in the spinal fluid helps to diagnose this condition.

Treatment with ACTH (corticotrophins) may be helpful in acute manifestations of this disease and is especially helpful in the treatment of eye involvement (retrobulbar neuritis). There is no other specific treatment for this disease. Efforts to maintain function and use of the limbs are promoted by exercise programs. Rest and adequate nutrition are important. In many patients, periods of spontaneous remissions permit normal life pursuits. Eventually, severe neurological disorders, such as paralysis, and weakness as well as other complications of impaired central nervous function, develop.

Dementia

Physicians increasingly see patients with dementia, which simply means intellectual deterioration. The typical victim is in the early 70s and comes for a check-up at the insistence of his or her spouse or relative who has noticed a failing memory or unusual behavior. When an especially sensitive observer is available, it may be possible to elicit a history of irritability, inefficiency at work, or lack of interest in things that were ordinarily important in the patient's life. The memory loss is minimal at first and progresses slowly. It consists of loss of recent memory, which means that events of the remote past can easily be recalled but the patient cannot remember what happened only a few hours previously. What usually precipitates the visit to the doctor is an outstanding social gaffe, a brief period of confusion, or a problem in controlling the urine.

A careful medical history and physical examination are essential at this point because many different disease processes can cause dementia. Sometimes there are findings of a disease that involves systems other than the brain: certain hormonal disturbances, pernicious anemia, some rare vitamin deficiencies, syphilis of the brain, a specific form of liver disease, or long-term use of bromides. A number of central nervous system diseases are associated with dementia, including Huntington's chorea and several rare degenerative diseases. A brain tumor, brain injury from a clot due to an accidental blow to the head, arteriosclerosis of the brain, and chronic intoxication with certain drugs, may all be present with the clinical picture of dementia. A depressive reaction may initially also be indistinguishable from dementia. The exact diagnosis is extremely important, since many of these conditions are curable.

The most common cause of dementia is atherosclerosis, or narrowing of the blood vessels that bring oxygen and glucose to the brain, which may result in diffuse death of brain cells. The higher cortical cells responsible for intellectual functions are most susceptible to vascular damage. This tragic state can occur in younger persons in a disease called presenile dementia. The victim of this condition is usually in his early 50s when the intellectual deterioration begins, and it is usually first manifested by difficulties in his work. The clinical course is similar to those cases of dementia associated with vascular disease.

As the condition advances, the patient becomes careless of his or her appearance and personal habits. Judgment becomes impaired. The patient may have no interest in food and begin to lose weight. Memory becomes poorer, and events of only a few minutes before may be forgotten. The patient may get lost even in his own neighborhood or tend to wander around aimlessly. Sadness and laughter may alternate within a few minutes of each other. The dementia progresses, and the patient may lose control of his urine and of stools and finally may spend all his time in bed. His nutrition usually worsens, and pneumonia or some other infection often is the final event.

A few early cases have shown improvement after an operation (ventricular shunting) that drains off fluid from the normal cavities inside the brain. However, since results are unpredictable and complications are very common, this operation offers little help to the vast majority of persons with dementia. No satisfactory treatment is available, and at the moment no hopeful prospects are in sight. Custodial care often becomes necessary. As medical science improves life expectancy and our older population increases, a major social problem is developing concerning the care of these unfortunate persons.

Disorders of the Peripheral Nerves

In ordinary conversation, "nerves" and "nervous" generally refer to tension or anxiety, as we will discuss in another section of this book. However, when a doctor uses the word "nerve" in a technical sense, he is referring to a specific anatomical structure.

Our nervous systems can be divided into central and peripheral systems. The brain and the spinal cord make up the central nervous system. The peripheral nervous system consists of many nerves that connect the central nervous system with all parts of the body. The peripheral nerves are like telephone wires that bring messages in both directions between the central nervous system and our organs and tissues. Nerves vary in size and length. The typical nerve in a leg or arm, the median nerve in the forearm, for example, looks like a piece of cooked thin spaghetti.

If a nerve is cut in two, a number of effects are noted. Sensation is lost in the area supplied by that particular nerve. In other words, all the feeling is gone in that area. You could stick a pin into the skin and the victim would not feel it, or you could pinch or burn or freeze the skin without any discomfort resulting. The muscles supplied by the nerve that was cut would be unable to receive the message from the brain to contract, and those muscles would be paralyzed, totally useless.

As an illustration, let us see what happens when the median nerve is severed just below the elbow. This could happen in an automobile accident or from a stab wound. The ability to feel touch, pain, heat, or cold is decreased to some extent in the skin of the thumb and two-thirds of the palm on the thumb side of the hands and is completely lost over the last inch or so of the index and middle fingers. Sensation is decreased rather than totally lost in the larger area of supply because there is overlapping with some branches of nearby nerves. The victim will be unable to bend his thumb or to move the thumb to touch one of his other fingers with it. His grip will be weakened, as will flexion and turning outward of the wrists. He will not be able to turn his forearm so that the palm faces downward. After a time the large muscle at the base of the thumb will shrivel from non-use, and the hand will look like that of an ape, with all five fingers in the same plane, instead of with the thumb being at an angle to the other fingers. These effects can be minimized by surgical treatment. The severed nerve edges can be sewn together. Maximum recovery after such repair of a nerve cut near the elbow takes about a year.

A nerve may be injured but not cut through, as in an injury that compresses the nerve or one that causes inflammation and swelling in the tissues near the nerve and consequent pressure on the nerve itself. Some of the nerve fibers may be damaged and others spared. The effects on the patient depend on which fibers are involved. Besides loss of sensation and muscle power, another symptom of nerve injury is pain. This occurs when the nerve is irritated, as when it is compressed rather than completely severed. The fibers that carry pain are not destroyed (or loss of sensation would result, as we have seen) but rather stimulated, so that the patient feels pain that seems to originate in the area of supply of that nerve.

Inflammation of a nerve is called *neuritis*. There are a number of different causes, and the symptoms depend not only on the cause but also on which nerves or fibers within those nerves are involved, how severe the damage is to those fibers, and how quickly or slowly the disease process acts. We are going to describe several common types of neuritis.

Diabetic Neuritis

Neuritis is a common complication of diabetes mellitus, usually occurring in patients over 50 years of age, especially when control of the blood sugar has been poor. Inflammation of any nerve can occur, and a multitude of effects are possible, including paralysis of motion of one eye, diarrhea (from inflammation of the nerves to the bowels), and severe pain in one small area of the body.

The most common form of diabetic neuritis involves small nerve branches in the hands and feet. Numbness and tingling in the feet and lower legs are usually the earliest complaints, from inflammation of the sensory fibers of the nerves in these areas. The hands may also be involved. Pain is not common in these cases. Muscle weakness in the feet and hands is usually mild, but occasionally the weakness is worse than the numbness and tingling. On physical examination, areas of decreased sensation can be found in the toes and fingers, and the muscle reflexes that the doctor tests are decreased or absent. Strict regulation of the blood sugar is the treatment, and relief of symptoms over a period of a number of months is the rule.

Bell's Palsy

The facial nerve is called a motor nerve because it supplies the muscles of the face but not the sensation of the skin of the face. There is one facial nerve on each side that activates all the muscles of expression on that side. Inflammation of one facial nerve is a fairly common occurrence. The cause is not certain, but patients with this problem have often been in a draft of wind against that side of the face a day or two previously. As the inflamed nerve swells, it is squeezed by the walls of the narrow opening of the skull through which it passes, and the resulting damage causes a paralysis, or palsy, of the muscles it supplies on that side of the face. This is called Bell's palsy.

The victim is unable to close that eye, that corner of the mouth droops, and the normal skin folds and creases are smooth. Saliva drools from the affected side of the mouth.

Fortunately, nature heals the condition completely within a few weeks in 80 percent of cases. Cortisone treatment may decrease the small percentage of cases of permanent residual paralysis.

Trigeminal Neuralgia

The trigeminal nerve supplies sensation to the face, and like the facial nerves, which supply the muscles, there is one for each side. The three branches of the trigeminal nerve supply the upper, middle, and lower parts of the face. Trigeminal neuralgia, also called tic douloureux, is a disease whose cause is unknown, characterized by spasms of pain in one of the branches of the trigeminal nerve on one side of the face. The pain is extremely severe and lasts only for a few seconds or minutes at a time. It may occur as often as every two or three minutes for several weeks before spontaneously subsiding. Sometimes talking or chewing or touching the face triggers off a burst of pain.

Several medications seem to cause improvement, but

sometimes the pain is so severe that it is necessary to inject or even cut the involved branch of the trigeminal nerve. This causes a numbness in the area and is avoided whenever possible, since trigeminal neuralgia often disappears after a time.

Herpes Zoster

Another painful affliction of nerves is herpes zoster, commonly called the shingles. This is caused by the same virus that causes chickenpox and usually occurs in persons who have had chickenpox many years previously. The virus involves the sensory ganglion of one nerve, almost always on the trunk. Since it stimulates the pain fibers, it causes a severe burning sensation in a narrow band around one side of the body. A few days later red blotches are seen on areas of the skin supplied by the affected nerve, and soon small bubbles appear, containing a drop of clear fluid. As these bubbles in the skin break, they leave crusts, then heal completely. The pain is usually slower to subside, and in a few cases, especially in older persons, the pain persists for as long as a year or even two. This complication is called post-herpetic neuralgia.

Sciatica

One other form of neuritis, sciatica, refers to pain over the path of the sciatic nerve. Although sciatica is caused by a number of conditions, a common type is that due to compression by a herniated intervertebral disc of the roots that make up the nerve. This is described in the section on backache.

When the disc pinches the nerve, it causes pain in the lower back and down the back and outside of the thigh and calf. Tingling and numbness also often occur. Fortunately, the fibers to muscles are not usually badly damaged and a little weakness of the leg and foot is all that results, although occasionally we see "foot drop," that is, inability to extend the foot so that it flops downward.

Treatment depends on the cause of sciatica.

Symptoms you should know about:

Symptoms of disease of the nervous system are often so obviously serious that medical help is sought as soon as they occur, as in the sudden paralysis due to a stroke. Occasionally symptoms appear so insidiously that they are dismissed as unimportant, and persons adapt to **chronic headache, dizziness, visual disturbances, hearing loss, tremor, a memory defect, personality change, and localized weakness or numbness,** and do not seek medical help until long after their onset. **A convulsive seizure,** although dramatic, is of brief duration, and is often ignored because the subject feels well afterward. Sometimes persons with obvious neurological disease are unable or unwilling to recognize that they are sick, because impaired judgment may result from brain damage. All these problems may be symptoms of curable nervous system disease.

PSYCHIATRIC ILLNESSES 14

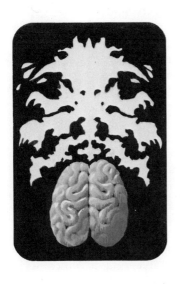

Medical specialties often are arbitrary divisions of fields of interest. People and diseases simply do not always fit into neat packages. Nowhere is this more obvious than in the patient with psychological symptoms or a psychological disease.

In the first place, physical illness may produce psychological symptoms, such as the depression that accompanies most serious illnesses, or the odd thinking and strange behavior seen with certain brain tumors. Secondly, a psychological conflict or illness may cause or aggravate physical symptoms or organic disease. The classic example of this situation would be a so-called psychosomatic condition, such as a peptic ulcer brought on by tension-producing circumstances at work. And, finally, patients with psychological disease may develop an unrelated physical illness; neurotic or psychotic persons do get pneumonia or cancer, or any other sort of organic condition. Because of these relations between psychological and physical illness, every doctor must be something of a psychiatrist.

A *psychiatrist* is a doctor of medicine who specializes in the diagnosis and treatment of mental and emotional illnesses. A *psychologist* is not a medical doctor, but rather one who has studied mental processes, both normal and abnormal. A *clini-*

cal psychologist works in the medical field, often helping the psychiatrist make a diagnosis through his expertise in psychological testing. Psychologists, by virtue of their knowledge of mental processes, sometimes counsel troubled people and even engage in psychotherapy, a field more usually dominated by the psychiatrist. *Psychotherapy* means treatment by talking with patients, as distinguished from the use of drugs, electroshock, surgery, or other physical measures.

Psychotherapy originated in psychoanalysis, which has been defined as "a psychologic theory of human development and behavior, a method of research, and a system of psychotherapy originally described by Sigmund Freud." Psychiatrists who employ the techniques of psychoanalysis are called psychoanalysts, or more popularly, analysts.

The main illnesses a psychiatrist sees are neuroses and psychoses. These are not always easily differentiated. Neuroses are illnesses thought to be caused by emotional conflicts, whereas psychoses are mental illnesses whose causes are unknown. The former are characterized by disordered feelings, while the latter are characterized by disordered thinking. According to Freud, "Neurosis does not deny the existence of reality, it merely tries to ignore it; psychosis denies it and tries to substitute something else for it." An old medical saw has it that neurotics are always building castles in the sky and psychotics live in castles in the sky. Feeling and thinking are so intertwined that there is some overlap in these two great classes of psychiatric disorders.

The term "nervous breakdown" is not a technical medical one, and it really has no well-defined meaning. It is most used to refer to an acute disabling psychological condition, and probably most nervous breakdowns are episodes of a suddenly worsened neurosis or psychosis.

Patients are sometimes reluctant to be referred to psychiatrists. Even in this enlightened age, many people attach a certain shame to any illness not obviously caused by "physical" factors. Some think that symptoms of a psychological illness are imagined or even faked by the sick person. In fact, persons with psychological illness may suffer as acutely as those with any other disease, and are as helpless to cure themselves. Well-meaning advice to "snap out of it" is about as effective for the patient with an anxiety neurosis as it is for the person with pneumococcal pneumonia. The patient with psychological problems needs a psychiatric consultation as much as the man with a broken leg needs an orthopedist, who is more capable of treating it because of his special training and experience in that field.

Neuroses

Within the category of neuroses there are several different sorts of illness. Depressive reactions and anxiety reactions are the most common and are discussed in greater detail later. *Anxiety neurosis*, where a feeling of nervousness is the predominant symptom, can be considered the simplest form of neurosis. The other neurotic reactions (described just below) reflect the way an individual handles his anxiety.

A *conversion reaction* means that unconscious thoughts or desires that are unacceptable to a person's conscious mind are converted to a dysfunction of skeletal muscle or one of the special senses. This sort of neurosis is also called *hysteria*, a term derived from the Greek word for uterus, because it was thought in ancient times that the disease was caused by a woman's uterus wandering about within her body. Conversion reactions are not common compared to other forms of neurosis. A classic example might be a teen-aged girl whose right hand is paralyzed because of guilt about masturbation. Cases of hysterical blindness and deafness are sometimes seen in young soldiers.

A *phobic reaction* is a specific fear without any reasonable basis. Common examples are fear of closed spaces (claustrophobia), fear of heights (acrophobia), fear of dirt and germs (mysophobia), fear of cats (ailurophobia), and even fear of the number thirteen (trisaidekophobia). According to psychiatric theory, the phobic reaction is a substitute fear for an actual fear or real responsibility in his life that the patient is unable to face.

Obsessive-compulsive reactions refer to constantly intruding stereotyped thoughts or to repetitive actions such as abnormally frequent hand-washing or complicated unvarying rituals that must be performed before the person can go to sleep. Many normal persons have minor obsessive-compulsive tendencies. The necessity to count all the panes in a window or tiles in a ceiling, or similar components of a pattern, is a common compulsion. We are familiar with the person who must close the open door, pick up a single scrap of paper from a clean floor, or rearrange the fork out of place at the table. Sometimes these compulsions can dominate a person's life;

many a woman spends all her hours cleaning and recleaning an immaculate house and feels nervous if she doesn't do so.

A *dissociative reaction* is a dramatic form of neurosis in which the patient mentally takes himself out of an unbearable emotional experience. He may temporarily seem not to know where he is, or what is going on about him. People around him may think he is drugged, or psychotic, because of his obvious separation from his surroundings. When he comes out of this fugue state, he has no memory for what occurred during that time. The total loss of memory (amnesia), which comic-strip and movie writers find convenient, is an example of a type of dissociative reaction.

Hypochondriasis is a neurosis, although today doctors recognize that this condition may represent the bodily expression of a depression. The hypochondriac usually has a long history of concern about his or her health. As a child he was often overprotected, and his every minor illness was a matter of grave concern. These patients complain of pain, usually in the head, chest, or abdomen, for which no cause can be found, and no amount of reassurance by the doctor can give relief. They will eventually have almost every x-ray and test known to the medical profession but always to no avail. These unfortunate persons go from doctor to doctor, but their quest for help is always in vain. They almost seem to enjoy narrating their medical adventures and to take pride in telling how their case has stumped the most prestigious specialist's diagnostic acumen. Actually diagnosis is usually not difficult, but treatment is as frustrating to the doctor as the disease is to the patient. When depression is an important part of the illness, drug therapy may be helpful. Minor psychotherapy is helpful when goals are kept modest; a sympathetic doctor can often keep these persons functioning in spite of their pains.

Psychoses

Psychoses are either organic or functional. In the former group, the cause is physical damage to the brain, such as from a syphilitic infection or impaired blood supply due to blockage of the arteries to the brain. In the latter group the cause is unknown at present. Occasionally it is difficult to distinguish a functional psychosis from an organic brain condition, but usually there are differences in the symptoms; even where the exact cause is not obvious, it is usually possible to tell whether a psychotic person is suffering from brain damage.

There are two major forms of functional psychosis: the manic-depressive psychosis and schizophrenia. Manic depressive psychosis is known as an affective psychosis, indicating that the disorder is primarily one of affect or mood. Schizophrenia, on the other hand, is basically a disorder of thinking.

The signs and symptoms of *manic-depressive* psychosis are so many and so varied that the famous French psychiatrist Kraeplin took 206 pages of his book to describe them! He was the first to recognize, in the last years of the nineteenth century, that all these different clinical pictures had some fundamental features in common, that persons with one form may develop another, and that all these cases had a similar prognosis. The least common form is the so-called circular or cyclic type, in which the patient suffers from alternating phases of mania and depression. Some patients may have only the manic phase, and the majority suffer only from the depressive phase.

Those who are prone to develop a manic psychosis are usually outgoing, breezy, brash, energetic persons. A mild degree of mania is called hypomania and is characterized by talkativeness, apparently boundless energy and self-confidence, much activity of all sorts, uninhibited speech and action, aggressiveness, boisterousness, and inability to tolerate routine. If the condition progresses to actual mania, all these traits are exaggerated. The person seems bursting with joyous excitement; he talks rapidly, jumping from one subject to another with bewildering speed; he can't sit still; he is in constant action, singing, shouting, running about, and seeming never to sleep. This goes on and on with unflagging energy. Paranoid ideas may develop, but hallucinations do not occur. The patient ignores injuries and infections, forgets to eat or drink, and if untreated may literally wear himself out.

Electroshock treatments are effective for the manic state but cause mental confusion and are used only as an emergency measure. Drugs which often control hypomanic or manic behavior are available for acute situations. A chemically simple drug, lithium carbonate, is very effective on a long-term basis but requires careful supervision because of possible toxic effects.

The depressive phase is much more common. Mild cases may often not be recognized as illness. When the condition is severe, the patient's mental and physical activities may be profoundly slowed and even progress to stupor. Psychotic depression is the commonest cause of suicide. Depression, both neurotic and psychotic, is discussed in greater detail later in this chapter.

The person with *schizophrenia* is usually recognized as such in late adolescence or early adulthood, but occasionally the diagnosis is first made later in life. Although many theories have been proposed and an enormous amount of research has been carried out over many years in this field, the cause remains completely unknown. External stress is not a cause of schizophrenia. The incidence in the U.S. Army is a remarkably steady two cases per thousand men each year, regardless of war or peace, and not related in any way to the patient's assignment. In other words, in the Army, schizophrenia is equally likely to occur in troops in the least stressful, safest, and easiest job as it is in those under the most arduous combat conditions. There is a wide variation in the severity of the disability due to schizophrenia; some persons may work daily and not be recognized to have this disease, while others are totally disabled and exist for many years in the back wards of psychiatric hospitals.

The symptoms vary from case to case. Several patterns may recur, but there is great overlapping within these clinical types.

Simple schizophrenia is characterized by withdrawal. These persons have little regard for social pressures and don't seem to "get involved." They drift along aimlessly, oblivious to those around them. Many tramps, vagrants, and prostitutes are simple schizophrenics.

Hebephrenic schizophrenic patients are silly, often giggling for no apparent reason. They seem to be in their own little world and have frequent hallucinations and delusions. Personality disintegration proceeds to the point where their emotional responses are shallow and their speech incoherent.

Probably the commonest variant is *paranoid schizophrenia*, in which the patient harbors delusions of persecution. He may think there is an organized conspiracy directed against him to harm or influence him. The victim often hears voices, usually threatening him, calling him vile names, and accusing him of obscene practices. These persons often go to doctors with bizarre physical complaints. Their emotional responses may be inappropriate, and they are usually suspicious and often unpleasant persons to be around.

Catatonic schizophrenia is characterized by a disorder of movement in which the victim maintains odd postures for long periods of time, immobile and seemingly unaware of his surroundings. He remains mute, ignores the normal calls of nature, even refusing to eat and drink. This state may be succeeded by catatonic excitement, with overactivity, sleeplessness, and finally exhaustion. As sick as they seem, these patients have a fairly favorable outlook for recovery.

Most psychiatrists recognize *pseudoneurotic schizophrenia* as a clinical type in which persons have a multitude of symptoms that seem to be neurotic but in such severe degree and enormous multitude that it is obvious that there is serious personality disorganization and loss of contact with reality.

Schizo-affective disorder is characterized by mood upsets, usually with depression, and resembles manic-depressive psychosis but with an added severe thinking disorder.

Many patients don't fit into any of these categories, and the term *undifferentiated type* is sometimes used to label such a schizophrenic person.

Tremendous advances in drug therapy of schizophrenia have been made in recent years, and several sorts of antipsychotic medications are now available. Various sorts of phenothiazines (including Thorazine, Mellaril, Haldol, Stelazine, etc.) are useful in even seriously ill schizophrenics. Skillful use of such drugs has resulted in an impressive decrease in the number of psychotic persons who require hospitalization. The treatment of schizophrenia usually requires a specialist in psychiatry.

Anxiety

Anxiety is a universal experience; everyone feels anxious at some time. The physical response to fear is the same as that which we feel in anxiety. When faced with danger our bodies react in many ways, and the effects are in proportion to the degree of danger. A person in an extremely perilous situation may show the following changes: his heart rate quickens, his blood pressure increases, his breathing becomes more rapid, the pupils of his eyes become larger, his skin is pale, cool, and covered with sweat, the hairs on his skin become erect, and he experiences a feeling of fear. Just the anticipation of danger, even when the threat fails to materialize, may cause a similar reaction and feeling. When the same sort of apprehension is felt, with or without the bodily changes, in a subject who is not in any peril and who does not recognize any external threat, we call this sensation anxiety.

Although everyone has experienced anxiety, many people live with this unpleasant sensation most of the time. They constantly feel tense, apprehensive, and ill at ease. If you ask them why they are tense, they will answer honestly that they don't know. These people are usually called nervous. Where anxiety is a constant or regularly recurring symptom that interferes with the activities of normal living, that person is said to have an *anxiety neurosis*. Of course, some degree of anxiety is present in all neuroses and at times in perfectly normal people, so the diagnosis of anxiety neurosis is limited to those cases where the anxiety is the outstanding symptom. Many persons live with anxiety yet manage not to have any restrictions of their activities or talents; this is called a *chronic tension state*.

Symptoms.   Anxiety may cause a great variety of symptoms. It has been said that each person has his own characteristic way of feeling anxious. In anxiety, first of all, the subject feels "nervous," which is a sort of fearfulness and a sense of uneasiness. Increased muscle tension may cause tremor, an unsteady voice, weakness, or aching and stiffness in various large muscles. Cardiovascular signs and symptoms include heart palpitations, fast pulse, increased blood pressure, lightheadedness, faintness, and either flushing or paleness of the skin. The gastrointestinal tract is involved and the anxious person may lose his appetite, become nauseated, and even vomit; abdominal distress is common, often called "butterflies in the stomach," and diarrhea is also frequently present. The hands and feet may become cold and moist ("clammy"), breathing is rapid or irregular, there may be frequency of urination, and sleep can be disturbed. Some unfortunate persons with an anxiety neurosis may have most of these symptoms, but most anxious persons have only a few of these.

What causes anxiety? The theory now held by practically all doctors is that anxiety is an expression of an unconscious emotional conflict. The conflict is between elemental urges which demand gratification and the conscience which recognizes that gratification would entail guilt or other undesirable consequences. An example is anxiety that results from the conflict between a sexual desire and the restrictions of society that make its expression impossible. In fact, probably more common emotional conflicts originate in nonsexual hostility or other aggressive drives that cannot be fulfilled because of social or other practical reasons. It must be emphasized that this conflict takes place at an unconscious level, and the person with the conflict is not aware that it is taking place. It is common for a "nervous" person (one who is experiencing anxiety) to blame his or her tension on an external problem, when in reality an entirely different emotional conflict is the cause. The following case is an example:

A forty-year-old man was seen because of severe anxiety of several months' duration. He felt that there was nothing that could be done about it because it was caused by concern over his wife's incurable neurologic disease, which confined her to a wheelchair and bed. She had been disabled for many years, but she was fully capable sexually, since they had had a child two years previously. Further questioning revealed that his anxiety had arisen since the frequent, prolonged visits of his best friend to his wife, visits ostensibly prompted by the charitable motive of visiting the sick. It seemed evident that the patient's anxiety was due to unconscious jealousy and hostility toward the friend.

Treatment. What can be done to alleviate anxiety? Theoretically, removal of the unconscious emotional conflict would seem to be the most effective means of treatment. However, this is seldom practical. Yet much can be done to improve the lot of these people.

First of all, the doctor must reassure the patient that although it is subjectively very disturbing the anxiety itself is not a reflection of serious organic disease. This requires a careful medical examination to be sure that such disease is in fact not present. Sometimes diagnosis is not easy, since anxiety can produce symptoms similar to those of hyperthyroidism, heart disease, abdominal problems, or even cancer, and occasionally x-rays and laboratory tests may be required to be sure. Equally important is the reassurance that anxiety does not lead to psychosis; many very tense persons say that they are afraid they are going to lose their minds. When the difference between emotional and mental disease (neurosis and psychosis) is explained, this simple reassurance alone often diminishes the anxiety.

Second, commonsense measures to ensure healthful living are helpful. Regular meals, adequate rest, avoidance of excessive amounts of stimulants such as coffee and alcohol, and proper exercise all contribute to emotional as well as physical well-being.

Third, changes in the patient's environment may be desirable to avoid obviously stressful situations. Changing jobs or moving to a new residence is occasionally necessary to eliminate otherwise unavoidable serious problems. In general, these measures are not as successful as one could hope, and major changes in life style are not to be undertaken without exhausting all other possible avenues of reducing anxiety. Counseling is often desirable when anxiety seems related to domestic problems, financial difficulties, spiritual worries, etc. The physician is often helpful here, but sometimes clergymen, marriage counselors, social workers, school officials, or lawyers may be more effective.

When anxiety is of long duration and disabling, psycho-therapy is often beneficial. In severe cases, this should be undertaken only with a specialist trained in this field, a psy-chiatrist. In some patients, the unconscious conflicts that produce anxiety can be uncovered and dealt with, offering considerable relief of suffering and increase in productivity.

Finally, anxiety can be treated with medications. Sedatives and tranquilizers are commonly used to help those persons with anxiety severe enough to bring them to a doctor. A number of drugs are available that effectively reduce anxiety; and in proper doses, some of these are quite safe.

Just how widespread anxiety is can be inferred from the fact that in 1973 the most commonly prescribed drug in America was the tranquilizer Valium (diazepam). Fifty-seven million prescriptions were written that year for Valium, and one out of every ten adults in America took the drug at one time or another. The third most commonly prescribed drug was Lib-rium (chlordiazepoxide hydrochloride), a similar tranquilizer with almost the same actions and uses. Incidentally, even larger percentages of the population used Valium in most of the countries of Europe, reaching a high of 17 percent in France and Belgium.

Although some persons may experience drowsiness with any of the tranquilizers, this side effect is not too common with Valium and Librium, and many persons tolerate sedative doses of drugs that in larger amounts are actually used to induce sleep. Psychological dependence upon tranquilizers can develop, although actual addiction is not a serious problem except with the barbiturates. Side effects may occur with any drug, of course, but in the case of tranquilizers these undesirable effects are usually related to the dose. Simply cutting back the amount may remove the side effect, while the medications still often help the anxiety. In using these drugs, it must always be remembered that although they alleviate the distress associated with anxiety, they have no effect upon the emotional conflicts that are at the root of the problem. Continued long-term use is usually undesirable, although it may be necessary in some cases of anxiety neurosis.

Depression
Depression is the most common condition many physicians encounter in their practice. Some degree of depression accompanies all serious illnesses, though frequently depression is the only illness present. A depression may be neurotic in origin, that is, it may be a reaction caused by an emotional conflict, or it may be psychotic, in which case the depression is usually more profound and can be accompanied by a loss of contact with reality, to some degree.

The classic picture of a full blown depression is relatively uncommon, as compared to the depression symptoms that we see literally every day. But let us talk about the extreme first. The severely depressed patient looks unhappy, does not show any expression except that he may weep for no obvious reason, is quite inactive, and has little to say. Frequently he or she will not care about personal appearance, and will be unshaven, unkempt, or sloppily dressed. The depressed person may just sit staring out the window all day and even not get out of bed. When asked questions, he may not answer or may mumble briefly, and will not begin a conversation or say anything spontaneously. Such a patient is convinced that life is not worth living, and, if he had the energy, he would kill himself. He has feelings of worthlessness or vague guilt and sometimes ideas of persecution. Often such persons have the delusion that they have cancer or other incurable illness and that death is near. These tragic people have no hope for the future. They say that they feel blue, and friends and relatives can see this in the way they appear and act. A severe depression may be obvious even to a total stranger.

Doctors know that an underlying depression may cause sickness in persons who don't look or act depressed, and they are alerted for this in the patient who complains of being tired all the time or who has headaches, poor appetite, trouble sleeping, a bad memory, or trouble concentrating. Less severe depressions may not be obvious at all and not be suspected by the people around the afflicted person or even by the doctor he may consult for some vague feeling of not being well.

Sleep disturbances are common; the patient may either have insomnia or sleep too much. A typical pattern of insomnia is that of early morning awakening and inability to fall asleep again. The appetite may become poor, and weight loss is common; but some depressed patients eat more and gain weight. The change in sleeping and eating habits is a clue to the doctor that the person may be depressed. Another common complaint is a changed pattern of bowel movements, usually resulting in constipation but sometimes in diarrhea. Other common physical symptoms are headaches and fatigue. Typically the patient feels tired even on arising in the morning, but improves as the day goes on and feels best in the evening. He often has difficulty in concentrating, and his attention span may be so shortened that watching television or reading a book is no longer enjoyable. Similarly, memory may be impaired especially for recent events; he may remember events of 20 years ago but be unable to recall what he had for breakfast. These patients feel unhappy, hopeless, and unwanted. Crying spells are frequent, even for no obvious reason.

As the symptoms of a depression develop and progress, there may be a concomitant increase in anxiety, and feelings of tension or nervousness may predominate. These can become so severe that psychiatrists often see patients with what they diagnose as "agitated depression."

What causes a depression? Unfortunately, there is no single answer to this question, but we do know some of the circumstances that seem to precipitate such an illness, and psychoanalysts have worked out a theoretical basis for this condition. There are also biochemical abnormalities that are associated with depression but do not necessarily cause it, which we shall discuss when we talk about treatment.

A simplified psychological explanation for a depressive reaction is that a depression results when there is a discrepancy between what a person is in his own eyes and what he thinks he ought to be. Psychoanalysts have a more elaborate explanation, based on the model of a *grief reaction*. The grief reaction following the death of a loved person is in many respects similar to a depressive reaction. When we love someone, we identify with that person, that is, we unconsciously incorporate part of that person's personality into our own, and we pattern ourself after the one we love. All human love relations are thought to contain some aspect of ambivalence, with an element of hate unconsciously mixed with the love. When a loved one dies, because of the identification and ambivalence, there are two psychologic effects. First, the mourner feels the loss as though part of himself had died. Secondly, he feels an unconscious guilt that in turn generates the feeling that the mourner should die or will die as punishment for the loved one's death. The loss plus guilt are reflected in sadness, helplessness, bitterness, retardation of psychic processes (the problems with memory and concentration mentioned above), and mental uneasiness, sometimes even with death wishes or other suicidal thoughts. Other processes of the body are affected, with changes in eating, sleeping, elimination, and so forth. Thus, the state of mourning can look very much like a depression.

Depression may begin for no obvious reason, or it may seem to stem from a significant happening in the patient's life. In the latter case, we call it a "reactive depression," implying that the depression is a reaction to an event. Some common examples of such situations are: death of, or separation from, a loved person, failure in a job, retirement, major surgery or serious illness, sudden assumption of overpowering responsibilities, and paradoxically, sudden success after strenuous efforts, such as a promotion at work. Some of the most severe cases are seen in women who have just given birth to a child, and the menopause is also a frequent occasion for depression. Of course these are merely immediate causes and not the complete cause, since most people handle such events successfully. All ages are susceptible, but middle age seems to be an especially vulnerable time. Conscientious, hardworking, self-sacrificing persons seem to be more than usually prone to depression as they approach old age.

Every seriously depressed person is a potential suicide, and most suicides in our society do occur in depressed persons. It has been said that suicide is most often a symptom or the last expression of a psychiatric disorder, not a free moral choice. The depressed phase of manic-depressive psychosis presents the greatest risk, with alcoholism in second place. Other mental illnesses, especially schizophrenia, may also predispose to suicide. Suicide has ranked tenth or eleventh as a leading cause of death in the United States for many years and may really be even more frequent, since self-destruction may appear accidental or may be deliberately concealed.

Any suicidal threat should be taken seriously. Most persons who kill themselves have threatened it or spoken about it before they actually perform the deed. An especially susceptible time is when a person appears to be recovering from a depression. It almost seems as though the degree of recovery gives the victim enough energy to finally carry out the suicidal thought.

Treatment. The treatment of depression is in many ways similar to that of anxiety, except that different sorts of drugs are used. Psychotherapy may be especially important in these people, given the problem of suicide as mentioned above. Severely depressed patients are best treated by the psychiatrist rather than by the family physician.

In the past few years, a new class of drugs has become available for the treatment of depression, called, appropriately enough, *antidepressants*. These medications are not stimulants and do not improve the mood of persons who are simply unhappy or dissatisfied with their life station. Their mode of action seems to depend upon the fact that in many depressed persons there is a depletion of certain normal chemicals, called amines, within the brain. Evidence for this is that some persons using reserpine for high blood pressure become depressed. Reserpine reduces the amount of amines in the brain, and this reserpine-induced depression can be reversed by administering another drug, called Dopa. Also, the amount of amines excreted in the urine has been observed to be decreased in depressed persons. Iproniazid, a drug that inhibits the normal removal of amines from nerve tissue and therefore increases the amounts of amines in the brain, is often an effective antidepressant. Imipramine, a different sort of effective antidepressant, increases the effects of amines (even though it does not increase the amount).

Research on the chemical reactions within the brain is important not only because it points out a way to treat depression but also because it may open up our understanding of emotional reactions. Many other facts have accumulated on the role of the amines in mood disorders, not all of them consistent with the simplified idea that the amount in the brain correlates with depression or elation. Much more work must be done in these promising areas.

Two types of antidepressant drugs are available for treatment. Drugs like iproniazid, called monoamine oxidase inhibitors, carry the larger risk of side effects. The other type, like imipramine, are called tricyclic antidepressants; they are in general similarly effective and safer to use. The trade names of the most commonly prescribed tricyclic antidepressants are Tofranil, Elavil, and Sinequan.

In general, these medications do not work quickly, and frequently no result is noted until the patient has been using them for two weeks or so. The dosage differs from person to person and must be worked out by trial and error. Side effects include dryness of the mouth, constipation, slowing of the urinary stream, low blood pressure, seizures, and rarely tremors and rigidity. Occasionally some persons react in an opposite manner than desired and become increasingly restless and agitated while using these medications. Those who do not experience these side effects or have only mild adverse reactions frequently have good results. Increased appetite and improved sleeping are the first good signs and then the mood improves and all symptoms are better. The duration of treatment cannot be foretold, but it is at least for a month or two after maximum benefit has been achieved.

Psychosomatic Medicine
When we speak of a psychosomatic illness, we mean one in which emotional problems play an important causative role. Research in the 1930s and the 1940s showed that certain personality traits were associated with certain illnesses, and it was theorized that these illnesses were caused by the emotional problems of those patients. Typical examples were duodenal ulcers, chronic ulcerative colitis, bronchial asthma, hives, high blood pressure, hyperthyroidism, and rheumatoid arthritis.

For example, it was found that patients with duodenal ulcers were often tense persons who had unconscious dependency needs, that is, they wished to be loved and cared for. However, at the same time, on a conscious level they were ambitious and wanted to be self-sufficient; in fact, they often were hard workers with a good record of success. The frustration of their dependency needs caused overactivity of the stomach and excessive secretion of the acid stomach juices, and this finally resulted in an ulcer.

The psychosomatic concept became very popular, and soon everyone was using the term. "Adelaide's Lament" from a hit Broadway musical was a humorous example of the overuse of the expression; poor Adelaide's frustrated marital ambitions were expressed in sneezing, and she proclaimed that she had a "psychosomatic cold." As doctors began to realize that there was an emotional component to almost all illnesses, the term was increasingly applied to more and more conditions, so that finally misuse and overuse blunted its meaning. The word "psychosomatic" is no longer used by most doctors.

Another reason for abandoning the term is that, paradoxically, it fostered ideas that were the exact opposite of the original concept. It seemed to mean that there was a psyche (mind) and a soma (body), and that they were two distinct entities reacting upon one another. Throughout history, philosophers have been preoccupied with the question of whether mind and body are separate things. Today doctors generally consider that this philosophic problem is not relevant and that mind and body are simply two different ways of looking at the same thing—a human being, who wouldn't be human without one or the other.

Although the expression "psychosomatic" has fallen into disfavor, some of the original ideas behind the concept were excellent, and much research has been carried out to show how our bodies react to external and internal pressures. Psychologists make a distinction between affect, which is the mental process that causes an emotion, and emotion, which is the feeling itself. A homely example of this distinction is the affect of embarrassment and the emotion of feeling embarrassed, often associated with a discharge of the autonomic nervous system to cause widening of the blood vessels in the skin of the face, visible to all as a blush. Actually, the words "affect" and "emotion" are often used interchangeably, since in practice they are indistinguishable. We will stick to "emotion," the word used in everyday life.

Emotions cause nerve activity in the cerebral cortex, the outer layer of the brain, which is so highly developed in human beings. The cells of the cortex transmit nerve impulses to the hypothalamus, a structure deep within the brain. The hypothalamus relays the nerve message back to other areas of the cortex and then to the autonomic nervous system. This system consists of nerves to tiny smooth muscles and glands over which we have no conscious control and which affect the eyes, blood vessels, skin, heart, gastrointestinal tract, and indeed all of our organs. This autonomic nervous discharge accounts for the bodily changes we have mentioned that may accompany anxiety. In addition, the hypothalamus controls the pituitary gland and the endocrine organs that make the hormones in our bodies. Thus emotions have many physical repercussions on our bodies, and long-continued activity of these mechanisms can even result in structural bodily changes, such as the duodenal ulcer mentioned above.

Normal Sleep and Sleep Disorders

Disturbances of the sleeping pattern occur commonly in depressed persons, as we have seen. Sleep disorders are such common problems and are of so much concern to the persons involved that we will consider the subject in more detail.

Babies spend most of their time asleep, and periods of wakefulness generally lengthen during childhood. Adults average approximately seven hours of sleep a day, but there is a wide variation in this from person to person, depending on habit, psychological factors, life style, and not yet understood individual differences. One person may seem to require nine or ten hours of sleep daily while another seems to get by with five. In general, women get about one hour more sleep per day than men do. There is no evidence that older people need more or less sleep than middle-aged or young adults.

During the 1960s considerable research was conducted on sleep in many centers throughout the world, but particularly in the United States. This activity developed from the exciting discovery that there are two distinct kinds of sleep, as determined by brain-wave studies. The electrical activity of the brain undergoes several changes as we pass from wakefulness into a relaxed state, then light sleep, then into a deep sleep. There are four stages of brain-wave changes during this first kind of sleep. After an hour or so of deep sleep, a fifth stage is seen, so different that it was originally called "paradoxic sleep," but now is usually known as REM sleep.

REM means "Rapid Eye Movement," so-named because of the most characteristic feature of this stage. This REM sleep is associated with very rapid brain waves, indicating a good deal of activity going on in the brain. During this sort of sleep, the eyes remain closed, and the subject is deeply asleep, but the eyeballs are moving rapidly and irregularly, the heart rate increases, the breathing becomes more rapid, more oxygen is used by the body, and more urine is formed. Most interestingly, dreaming occurs during this REM sleep. After a few minutes to a half hour, non-REM sleep appears again.

Similar cycles of 70 to 100 minutes succeed each other for the rest of the night. Most adults have between four and six cycles during each night's sleep. REM periods often lengthen with each cycle, and REM sleep makes up about 20 to 25 percent of the total sleep time. This means that normally from one fifth to one quarter of our time asleep is spent in dreaming, with our brain working quite busily.

If we are awakened during REM sleep, we will usually remember what we were dreaming about. If we awaken naturally as we come back to light sleep, we will feel refreshed and rested, even after only one or two cycles. However, if we are awakened during deep sleep, we will be groggy and feel we need more sleep even though we may have slept seven or eight hours. Persons who say they never dream probably always awaken from non-REM sleep.

Insomnia.   Insomnia means difficulty in falling asleep, frequent awakening during the night, or awakening too early and being unable to fall asleep again. The most frequent cause of insomnia is an emotional upset. The prevalence of long-term insomnia illustrates how frequently chronic depression is found among the general population. Any sort of psychic stimulation prior to bedtime may also keep one awake. The caffeine in coffee is a stimulant that prevents sleep for many perfectly normal people.

Besides getting less sleep, persons with chronic insomnia have a poorer quality of sleep with more time in light sleep and less time in deep sleep. Their heart rate is not as slow nor temperature as low, and they are more easily aroused from their sleep than persons who do not complain of insomnia. The percentage of REM sleep is neither decreased nor increased.

Many different sorts of drugs are used to promote sleep, including barbiturates (for example, phenobarbital, Seconal, Tuinal, and Nembutal), chloral hydrate, glutethimide (Doriden), fluorazepam (Dalmane), and others. This general class of drugs is called hypnotics. Studies in sleep laboratories where brain waves are constantly recorded show that hypnotics are quite effective in helping people fall asleep and stay asleep. However, after about two weeks of consecutive use, the great majority of hypnotic drugs lose their effectiveness; in fact, the only possible exception is Dalmane. With chronic drug use there is a decrease in REM sleep and also a marked decrease in deep sleep, so that the person spends most of the night awake or in light sleep. Even after these drugs are not working, patients who use them are reluctant to discontinue their use. The reason for this is that things are even worse for a time after stopping the hypnotic drug. Difficulty in falling asleep is especially severe, and the time in REM sleep becomes considerably increased, so that disturbing dreams are common during the period of drug-withdrawal insomnia. This disturbance of sleep and dream patterns makes the victim dependent on continued hypnotic drug use. Treatment of the underlying emotional problem is necessary if a longstanding insomnia is to be relieved.

Because of this problem, simpler measures are much preferred in inducing sleep. A hot bath is often relaxing enough so that people who would otherwise have insomnia are able to fall asleep easily. Many persons drink warm milk at bedtime, and some find that a small amount (one half to one ounce) of brandy is an effective sleep-inducer.

Hypersomnia. At the other end of the sleep spectrum are those persons who sleep too much—people with hypersomnia. These people are difficult to arouse, and when they waken they are often confused and groggy. Depression is the most common cause of this problem, just as it is in persons with insomnia. Rare causes of hypersomnia are damage to a certain brain center (which is often also associated with eating too much) and the shallow breathing seen in some grossly overweight persons.

Narcolepsy. Altogether different is the condition called narcolepsy, which is characterized by an irresistible need to sleep for a few minutes to a half hour and which occurs many times a day. No one knows the cause of this disease. Its victims are often embarrassed by suddenly falling asleep in public. Fortunately, certain stimulant drugs are quite effective in treating narcolepsy.

Night Terrors. Night terrors occur mostly in children, but grown-ups can also have them. They are characterized by awakening during the night with intense anxiety and fear, with trembling, pounding of the heart, and a cold sweat. The child (or adult) does not recall any bad dream and does not know what caused his terror. Night terrors usually occur fairly soon after falling asleep, during the first sleep cycle of the night. Frequently the victim does not awaken but observers can see the restlessness and obvious signs of fear. Children frequently outgrow this condition. Its cause is unknown.

Nightmares are different from night terrors in that they are commonly seen in all ages, come on in REM sleep, and the bad dream is remembered after awakening.

Sleepwalking.   It has been estimated that between one and six out of every hundred persons has walked in his sleep. This occurs during non-REM sleep, and the subjects have no memory for the episode after awakening, so that sleepwalking does not represent the acting-out of a dream. Episodes last from a few seconds to a few minutes. Various activities may be performed during the sleepwalking episodes, but none that require fine movements or careful coordination. This condition is usually associated with a psychological disturbance. Children outgrow it. Sleepwalkers do not tend to hurt themselves during the episode but seem to walk around furniture in the middle of the room almost as though they knew it was there. There is no special danger to awakening persons during this state, and the old wives' tale about inducing mental illness by awakening a sleepwalker is groundless.

Alcoholism

It is only in recent years that alcoholism has come to be regarded as a disease. In the past, most persons either ignored the problem completely or considered alcoholism to be a moral failing. "Drunk" jokes were part of every comedian's repertoire. But society has been forced to deal with alcoholism as a significant factor in unemployment, welfare costs, automobile and industrial accidents, and as an important cause of disability and death, as well as the source of untold suffering inflicted on these victims' families and associates. The courts have come to recognize alcoholism as an illness, and both the American Medical Association and the World Health Organization look upon it as a specific disease entity. Psychiatrists often see alcohol abuse as a symptom or complication of emotional or mental illness, but when the condition dominates the clinical picture, it is most practical to consider alcoholism as an illness in itself.

What is alcoholism?   Certainly, most people who use alcohol are not alcoholics, and even getting drunk on any specific occasion does not imply the illness we are talking about. Sometimes it is easy to recognize an alcoholic. It doesn't take much of a diagnostician to spot the disheveled old man, sprawled in a gutter on skid row and clutching a gallon bottle of wine, as an alcoholic. But even associates and friends may not know that the successful businessman, or lawyer, or suburban housewife is also an alcoholic who may be headed for the same deterioration. Almost everyone who has thought about it has his own definition of alcoholism. We will accept the following one offered by the AMA: "Alcoholism is an illness characterized by preoccupation with alcohol and loss of control over its consumption, such as to lead usually to intoxication if drinking is begun; by chronicity; by progression, and by tendency toward relapse. It is typically associated with a physical disability and impaired emotional, occupational, and/or social adjustments as a direct consequence of persistent and excessive use of alcohol."

The alcoholic may be male or female, black or white, rich or poor; he may live in the city or the country, be young or old, single or married. The cause of alcoholism is not known. It is probable that there is no single cause but rather that many factors combine to produce the condition.

Many organic theories have been proposed to explain why some persons become alcoholic. These include disorders of sugar metabolism, endocrine defects (hypothyroidism has had a recent vogue), deficiency of vitamins or minerals, allergy, and a biochemical or structural abnormality in the brain. None has ever been proved. It is certain that alcoholism is not hereditary.

There is a physiological element that partly explains the long-term nature and progression of the condition. Alcohol has a depressant effect on the brain. How strong this effect is and how long it lasts, are related to the amount of alcohol that is drunk and over how long a period of time it is consumed. The central nervous system depressant effect causes relief of tension, and decreases inhibitions, resulting in a relaxed and "loosened up" feeling. Large amounts quickly consumed can cause enough depression of nerve function to bring on drowsiness, sleep, unconsciousness, and even death. When the alcohol is metabolized by chemical reactions in the body, the depressant effect wears off and is succeeded by a rebound excitability in nerve tissue, roughly proportional to the degree and duration of the depressant effect. When severe, this excitability causes a sensation of unease or anxiety, and may even produce agitation and trembling. These discomforts, plus the "morning after" headache, guilt, and depression, can be temporarily helped by taking in more alcohol to get the pleasant nervous system depressant effect again. When this cycle is repeated over and over again, the relief from the after-effects becomes more necessary, and physical and psychological dependence develops.

There is some statistical evidence that sociological factors play a part in causing alcoholism. In some cultures or religious groups the use of alcohol is completely forbidden; members of these groups rarely become alcoholics. The average American community of our time has an ambivalent position concerning alcohol. Abstinent and permissive attitudes exist side-by-side. Guilt over drinking may dilute an artificial feeling of masculinity or sophistication attached to alcohol use. Where these illogical ideas about alcohol are present, alcoholism is a common problem.

Psychological factors are generally considered to be the most important in the development of alcoholism. The psychopathology is not certain, but it seems that the alcoholic is an emotionally immature or disturbed person who relies on the effects of drinking to relieve anxiety, depression, insecurity, hostility, and guilt that he cannot otherwise handle. Repeated use establishes the drinking of alcoholic beverages as a pattern of behavior.

Complications. Alcoholism ravages the human body. Gastritis, peptic ulcer, pancreatitis, fatty liver, and cirrhosis with all its complications occur in alcoholics. Many alcoholics die from liver disease, but even after cirrhosis has developed, it is impossible to say when the liver damage has passed the point of repair, so all persons with alcoholic cirrhosis should be encouraged to stop drinking alcohol. Sometimes patients who appear to be dying of liver disease can make complete recoveries after discontinuing the use of alcohol.

Alcohol may cause cardiomyopathy, or degeneration of the heart muscle. This leads to enlargement and irritability of the heart so that the heartbeat becomes irregular. Finally, congestive heart failure occurs and may prove fatal. However, just as in the case of cirrhosis, a complete recovery may follow discontinuing alcohol use.

As might be expected from what we said about the effect of alcohol on nervous tissue, a large number of neurologic disorders are associated with alcoholism. Peripheral neuropathy, or neuritis, causes numbness, crawling or pins-and-needles sensations, pains, weakness, and even paralysis of the extremities. Wernicke's disease is caused by deficiency of thiamine, one of the B vitamins, and occurs almost exclusively in alcoholics. It is characterized by paralysis of the eye muscles and disordered equilibrium, which interferes with walking and makes balance difficult to maintain. Mental symptoms are often associated with this condition, especially Korsakoff's psychosis, with a severe memory defect. Some neurologic complications of a prolonged drinking bout come on shortly after the spree is over; these include tremulousness ("the shakes"), hallucinations, convulsions ("rum fits" or "whiskey fits"), and delirium tremens (the "DT's").

This last is a dramatic and sometimes dangerous complication with a significant mortality rate. The condition begins suddenly with trembling, agitation, confusion, and signs of autonomic nervous system activity such as sweating, fever, rapid heart rate, and dilated pupils. Vivid hallucinations occur, especially visions of animals or insects. The victim is unable to sleep during the episode, which usually lasts two or three days and clears up with the arrival of a deep sleep. High fever and shock occur in the fatal cases. Fortunately, medical treatment is available, consisting of intravenous fluids, vitamins, measures to combat fever, sedation of a degree short of depressing brain function, and prevention and handling of complications.

Treatment. The treatment of alcoholism is often a frustrating experience for the patient, the doctor, and the patient's family, but it can also be an immensely rewarding one, resulting in the restoration of a human being to useful life. Despite repeated failures, it is imperative not to give up. The most hopeless-seeming cases may eventually be cured.

Initial treatment is often carried out in a general hospital, since a complication of alcoholism or a prolonged drinking bout is usually the event that bring patients to the doctor. The "drying out" is used to evaluate the patient's physical condition. Medical treatment of any abnormalities found is begun. When the drinking pattern has been interrupted, emergency problems corrected, and any necessary long-term medical treatment has been started, then a rehabilitation program is indicated. Some patients will be referred to psychiatric facilities, some to half-way houses that specialize in alcoholic problems, and many will be returned to their home and job with further measures arranged. Psychiatric treatment

Some Facts About Drinking

1. A one and one-half-ounce "shot" of whiskey contains 110 calories, and a 12-ounce can of beer 150 calories. You can get fat on alcohol!

2. The effects of alcoholic beverages depend on the amount of alcohol consumed, how fast it is taken in, previous drinking experience, body size, and psychological condition at the time of drinking.

3. The alcohol of beer, wine, scotch, bourbon, rye, gin, vodka, or liqueurs is all the same in the body. The flavor has nothing to do with the important effects. More concentrated drinks, such as straight whiskey or a dry martini, have more "kick" than a dilute drink, such as beer, because the equivalent amount of alcohol is drunk in a shorter time.

4. The average person can burn up about one-half ounce of pure alcohol per hour, or the rough equivalent of a little less than one highball, half a cocktail, or 12 ounces of beer.

5. Even one drink may affect your driving. If you are drinking, don't drive. Alcohol causes one half of all auto accidents in which the driver is killed.

6. There are at least 8 or 9 million alcoholics in the United States now. They live an average of 12 years less than nonalcoholics.

should be tailored to the particular patient. Formal individual psychotherapy is sometimes necessary and helpful. Family counseling may be desirable to repair a threatened marriage. The most effective psychotherapy for most alcoholic persons is group therapy with others who share the same problem. Religious, industrial, and labor union programs are available in some communities, and many have produced excellent results. One organization in particular must be mentioned as having successfully rehabilitated innumerable persons throughout the country—Alcoholics Anonymous. Almost every community has a branch of A.A., and usually it can be located by simply consulting the telephone book.

As with other diseases, prevention of alcoholism is much more likely to be effective in decreasing its human toll than treatment of already established cases. The "noble experiment" of Prohibition was foredoomed to failure. Except in certain restricted cultural atmospheres, total abstinence is totally impossible. Education of teenagers, promotion of a rational social attitude toward alcohol use, and detection and treatment of incipient cases give the most promise for decreasing the incidence of alcoholism.

Drug Abuse

"A desire to take medicine is perhaps the greatest feature which distinguishes men from other animals," said Sir William Osler. A drug is "any chemical agent that affects living protoplasm." This broad definition means that the term encompasses any substance that has an effect upon the body or mind. We will be concerned here with only a few drugs, those which produce changes in mood and behavior and have the potential for causing drug dependence. It is convenient to distinguish two sorts of drug dependence: habituation and addiction.

Habituation is a psychological rather than physical need for the drug to maintain an optimal state of well being. This need may vary in intensity from only a mild desire to such an intense craving that the habituated person spends most of his time thinking about the drug or trying to get it or actually using it. Drugs to which people become habituated are usually those that provide some relief from emotional tensions, that dull feelings of anxiety, and that produce a state of well being.

Addiction is a physical need for the drug. When an addicted person does not use or cannot get the drug, his body reacts with certain changes that cause distressing symptoms. This is called the withdrawal syndrome, and the actual symptoms vary with the nature of the drug involved. Withdrawal syndrome in someone who has been addicted to a narcotic for a long time may be so violent that it causes the death of the victim.

Usually, repeated use of the same amount of a drug causes less and less of an effect on the user, and he must take in larger amounts to produce the effects he got with his original dose. This phenomenon is called *tolerance*, and it is seen in both habituation and addiction. Habituation may precede addiction, so that in the early stages of drug abuse, the habit can be stopped without withdrawal symptoms, but after a longer period of use this is no longer true. Not all drugs produce tolerance or physical dependence.

The most commonly abused drugs in America now are marijuana, narcotics, sedatives, stimulants, and hallucinogens. Other substances are also abused, such as model airplane glue or other volatile solvents that can be sniffed to cause mental clouding, Jimson weed, and even large amounts of nutmeg. Alcohol abuse has already been discussed. Drug-dependent persons frequently abuse several different drugs. Doctors often encounter teenagers who take pills and capsules supplied by a "friend" without having any idea of what they contain or what effect they will produce. The problem of drug abuse continues to grow and is so widespread that the term "drug culture" has been coined to describe a group of people whose lives are dedicated to procuring and using drugs.

We do not know the ultimate cause of drug abuse. Both psychological and physical factors probably are involved. Mind-altering substances affect individuals differently, depending to a major degree upon the personality of the user. Tolerance may cause the need for increased amounts, and habituation may lead to addiction. The goal of avoiding withdrawal symptoms excludes almost all other goals from the addict's life.

Narcotics. It is impossible to know the extent of narcotic addiction in the United States, but unquestionably an enormous increase has taken place in the past ten years. In the middle of the 1960s there were approximately 60,000 known narcotic addicts in the United States, but by 1974, experts estimated that in New York City alone, more than 400,000 persons were addicted to opiate drugs.

A narcotic is a drug that relieves pain and induces sleep. This class of drugs is often called opiates, after opium, from which these agents are derived. Many drugs fall into this class—opium, morphine, heroin, codeine, meperidine (Demerol), and a host of others, many of which are used medically. The great majority of narcotic addicts take heroin. This is derived from morphine, but is about six times stronger. Heroin has no medical use, and the entire supply used in the United States is smuggled in. We will discuss the characteristics of heroin addiction and withdrawal here, since they are similar for all narcotics and differ only in degree.

The user buys heroin "on the street" from a "pusher" in a capsule or plastic bag which sells for between $2 and $10. It is always diluted ("cut") with milk sugar, quinine, and other materials; by the time it gets to the consumer there may be little of the heroin in the bag. The drug is taken intravenously "by the mainline," that is, by an injection into a vein, usually in the forearm.

The effects desired by persons who abuse heroin consist of a feeling of relaxation, elation, and the sensation of being in a pleasant dream. However, since the amount injected is unpredictable because of the dilution factor, there may be no effect at all or else undesirable toxic effects. When mild, these consist of nausea and vomiting. When severe, breathing is suppressed, the heart rate slows, the body temperature drops, and the victim slips into coma. Shock may develop, resulting in permanent brain damage or even death.

With frequent use of heroin, tolerance develops, requiring more and more of the drug for the same effect. Enormous amounts may be taken without toxic effects—many times the dose that would kill a normal person. The "high" feeling is generally lost as physical dependence develops, and the addict craves the drug just to approach feeling normal again.

Doctors have unfortunately become familiar with a number of medical conditions that are complications of narcotic use and addiction. Although heroin addicts may look perfectly normal, sometimes they are easily recognized by very small pupils of the eyes, frequent sniffing, flushed face, drowsiness, mental confusion, and needle marks and tracks of scarred veins in the arms and legs. A urine test can confirm the diagnosis of heroin use.

Malnutrition, personal neglect, and a host of infections are not unusual. Contaminated needles may spread infectious hepatitis, malaria, other blood infections, and even tetanus (lockjaw). Lung abscesses and infection of the heart valves are life-threatening complications of this sort of injection. Venereal disease is frequent among women addicts, a result of the prostitution necessary to earn the money to support the addiction. Tuberculosis and pneumonia are also common.

In an established addict, withdrawal symptoms begin after 8 to 16 hours without the drug. Yawning, sweating, running nose, and tearing eyes are the first symptoms, which progress over a period of hours. The victim cannot sleep and is restless and irritable. Nausea, vomiting, diarrhea, and pains in the abdomen, back, and legs occur on the second or third day. Alternating hot and cold feelings develop, and the restlessness becomes very severe. The symptoms reach a peak on the third or fourth day, then gradually subside over the next week or so. Insomnia, weakness, nervousness, and muscle aches may persist for several more weeks. Rarely a withdrawal syndrome may be so severe as to cause death with increasing fever and shock.

Cure of opiate addiction is possible. The relapse rate is high, and keeping the former addict from taking the drug again is the most difficult part of therapy. Substituting the drug methadone for the heroin is a widely known means of handling this problem. Although methadone is a narcotic, its effects are to decrease the craving for heroin and to blunt the "high" that heroin gives. It has undoubtedly helped many addicts to quit their heroin abuse and to resume normal lives. One objection to this form of treatment is that for it to be effective an indefinite program of use is required, and apparently few addicts can be taken off methadone completely without relapsing into heroin use. Special rehabilitation centers with group therapy support and individual psychiatric treatment are available in many communities.

Sedatives. Sedatives and tranquilizers have been mentioned in the discussion of anxiety. The most widely used sedatives belong to the chemical family of barbiturates. Some common trade names of barbiturates are Seconal, Nembutal, Luminal (which is better known by its generic name, phenobarbital), Amytal, and Butisol. They are called "downers" on the street and were also formerly known as "goof balls."

All these drugs are liable to cause physical addiction. These drugs are widely abused by all classes of society. Accidental overdose and suicide attempts lead to a significant number of deaths annually from barbiturates.

Stimulants. Stimulant drugs are called "uppers" and include amphetamines (Benzedrine), dextroamphetamines (Dexedrine), and methamphetamines (Methedrine). "Speed" is another slang name for these drugs.

A single dose of stimulant drugs can temporarily abolish fatigue and cause a sensation of alertness and well being. This effect leads to abuse by students who take them to keep awake while studying for and taking examinations, and by athletes, who call them "pep pills" and use them to enhance efforts in competitive sports. Stimulants also have physical effects, including elevation of the blood pressure, palpitations, rapid heart rate, headache, diarrhea, sleeplessness, and loss of appetite. This last effect accounts for their use in beginning a weight reduction program. Their stimulant effect is followed by a temporary depression.

Tolerance develops with repeated use, and psychological dependence occurs, although there is no withdrawal syndrome after stopping the drug. Prolonged use may cause liver damage and probably also brain damage. Cardiac arrhythmias and high blood pressure are potentially dangerous complications of long-term use of stimulants.

A large segment of the drug culture seeks "highs" from "speed trips," the intravenous use of amphetamines in large amounts. Some "speed freaks" inject the equivalent of 100 average doses into their body at one time. This causes an ecstatic "high" feeling of euphoria for a few hours, followed by depression as the stimulant wears off. Repeated speed trips carry a high risk of death.

Hallucinogens. Hallucinogens are drugs that alter sensations, producing distortion of time, space, and color perception, dreamlike experiences, vivid emotional responses of all sorts, delusions, and visual hallucinations. There are many naturally occurring drugs of this sort, also called psychedelics, found in cactus (mescaline), certain mushrooms, and plant seeds. The most potent is LSD, or lysergic acid diethylamide, produced in the laboratory from a fungus found on grain. In the middle 1960s, it was estimated that at least 4 percent of college students tried LSD at least once. Because of disastrous side effects, its use is decreasing.

The drug's effects are variable. When the emotional results

are terrifying, the delusions persecutory, and the hallucinations threatening, the user is said to have had a "bad trip."
Panic reactions may occur, and the victim become psychotic.
The psychotic state may disappear in a few days, but in some
cases it continues indefinitely. Days or even months after last
using LSD, a person may experience a "flashback," or a recurrence of a trip. Heavy users may develop brain damage, and
chromosomal changes occur, which theoretically may result in
deformed offspring.

Marijuana. Except for alcohol (and some would say coffee), the most commonly used mind-altering drug in America
is marijuana. Literally millions of Americans have tried
marijuana at least once. The drug is usually called grass or pot
by its users, and a marijuana cigarette is called a joint. Scientists know marijuana as "cannabis" from the hemp plant
that is its source. The active ingredient is tetrahydrocan-
nabinol, or THC.

There is a wide variation in the strength of marijuana
cigarettes. The flowering tops of the plant contain the most
THC, and the leaves have a lesser amount, while the stalks
and seeds have practically none. Marijuana brought in from
Mexico, Lebanon, or India is much stronger than that grown
in the United States. Wild-growing plants have less THC than
those especially planted and tended. Hashish ("hash") is
many times stronger than marijuana and consequently more
dangerous.

The immediate physical effects of smoking a joint are red-
dening of the eyes and cough (because of the irritant effect of
the smoke) and a rapid pulse; it makes some persons hungry
and others become drowsy. The desired psychologic effect is a
"high" feeling, which is a pleasant sensation of well-being,
freedom from tension, and a vague superiority. Distortions of
vision, hearing, and the sense of time often occur, and the
marijuana user may develop an unreal feeling, as though he is
dreaming. Mental performance may be impaired, but the person thinks he is functioning better than usual. Uncontrollable
laughing or crying sometimes occurs. Hallucinations are rare,
but can occur. These effects may last up to five to six hours if a
potent "joint" is used.

Marijuana does not lead to tolerance. Indeed, experienced
users can produce the desired effects with a smaller amount
than a novice. Marijuana causes habituation rather than addiction. Dependence is psychological rather than physical.

Continued regular use of marijuana may have adverse effects upon the user's personality. The habituated person, sometimes called a "pothead," tends to withdraw within himself, and to lose his ambition and drive. It is possible that there are harmful effects upon the brain, because poor memory and decreased mental sharpness are common among "potheads." Acute and chronic psychoses are seen in abusers of marijuana, but it is impossible to say whether the drug causes psychoses or whether psychotic or potentially psychotic persons are more likely to use drugs of any sort. At present it appears that the latter is more likely.

It has been said that the person who uses marijuana regularly may go on to the use of stronger drugs and become a narcotic addict. This belief arose because 85 percent of heroin addicts said that they had used marijuana before turning to "hard" drugs. However, only a small percentage of persons habituated to marijuana progressed to opium or heroin use. The psychological problems that create potheads are probably the same as those that lead to narcotic addiction, and so it is not surprising to hear that addicts have used other drugs.

Recent studies have shown that THC may be quite effective in preventing the nausea and vomiting associated with cancer chemotherapy.

Appendix I

Leading Causes of Death: United States, 1976*

Number	Causes of Death	Number of Deaths	Death Rate per 100,000 Population	Percent of Total Deaths
	All Causes	1,909,440	889.5	100.0
1	Heart disease	723,729	337.1	37.9
2	Cancer	377,312	175.8	19.8
3	Cerebral vascular disease	188,623	87.9	9.9
4	Accidents	100,761	46.9	5.3
5	Pneumonia	61,666	28.7	3.2
6	Diabetes mellitus	34,508	16.1	1.8
7	Cirrhosis of liver	31,453	14.7	1.6
8	Arteriosclerosis	29,366	13.7	1.5
9	Suicide	26,832	12.5	1.4
10	Diseases of infancy	24,809	11.6	1.3
11	Homicide	19,554	9.1	1.0
12	Emphysema	17,796	8.3	0.9
13	Congenital abnormalities	13,002	6.1	0.7
14	Kidney diseases	8,541	4.0	0.4
15	Blood stream infections	6,401	3.0	0.3
16	Others	246,087	114.7	12.9

*Source: Vital Statistics of the United States, 1976.

Appendix II

Recommended Schedule for Active Immunization

Age	Immunization
2 months	Diphtheria-Tetanus-Pertussis & Trivalent Oral Poliovirus
4 months	Diphtheria-Tetanus-Pertussis & Trivalent Oral Poliovirus
6 months	Diphtheria-Tetanus-Pertussis & Trivalent Oral Poliovirus
15-18 months	Measles, Mumps, Rubella (German measles)
18-24 months	Diphtheria-Tetanus-Pertussis & Trivalent Oral Poliovirus
4-5 years	Diphtheria-Tetanus-Pertussis & Trivalent Oral Poliovirus
14-16 years	Diphtheria-Tetanus—thereafter every 10 years.

Additional Immunizations

Travelers to Foreign Countries (must check with local Board of Health)

1. Typhoid vaccine
2. Cholera vaccine
3. Yellow fever vaccine
4. Typhus vaccine
5. Polio vaccine
6. Plague vaccine
7. Viral hepatitis immune serum globulin
8. Smallpox vaccine

Unusual Occupational Exposure

1. Smallpox vaccine
2. Plague vaccine
3. Rabies vaccine
4. Anthrax vaccine
5. Rocky Mountain spotted fever
6. Tularemia vaccine

Afterword

In the twentieth century, progress through greater understanding of health and disease has been enormous, derived from biochemistry, physiology, pharmacology, bacteriology, virology, immunology, molecular biology and psychology. Many infectious diseases have been eliminated or attenuated through preventive health measures, immunization, and the development of antibiotics. Refinements in blood banking technics and anesthesia have resulted in improvement in modern surgery. Organ transplantation and heart operations are now being performed. Newer forms of radiation treatment and the development of chemical agents and combinations of drugs have given remarkable results with certain types of cancer.

Even though the frontiers of medicine have been advanced more in this century than in all of past history, further improvements in life expectancy and the quality of life will require vast new knowledge to modify and prevent chronic degenerative diseases that appear to be produced at least partially from environmental factors in our relatively urbanized affluent society. In order for progress to continue, the general public must know as much as possible about Medicine, so that all can contribute to the decisions that our society must make in this field.

INDEX